LIVING
PAIN-FREE

ALSO BY DOREEN VIRTUE AND ROBERT REEVES, N.D.

Books

Nutrition for Intuition (available June 2015)
Angel Detox
Flower Therapy

Oracle Cards (divination cards and guidebook)

Flower Therapy Oracle Cards

ᕤ

ALSO BY DOREEN VIRTUE

Books/Calendar/Kits/Oracle Board

Awaken Your Indigo Power (with Charles Virtue; available March 2016)
Don't Let Anyone Dull Your Sparkle (available February 2016)
How to Get Your Life Back (with Brigitte Parvin; available January 2016)
Heaven's Messages for Us All (available October 2015)
Earth Angel Realms
Archangel Daily Messages 2015 Calendar
The Big Book of Angel Tarot (with Radleigh Valentine)
Angels of Abundance (with Grant Virtue)
Angel Dreams (with Melissa Virtue)
Angel Astrology 101 (with Yasmin Boland)
Assertiveness for Earth Angels
How to Heal a Grieving Heart (with James Van Praagh)
The Essential Doreen Virtue Collection
The Miracles of Archangel Gabriel
Mermaids 101
Flower Therapy (with Robert Reeves, N.D.)
Mary, Queen of Angels
Saved by an Angel
The Angel Therapy® Handbook

Constant Craving

The Yo-Yo Diet Syndrome

Losing Your Pounds of Pain

Audio/CD Programs

The Healing Miracles of Archangel Raphael

Angel Therapy® Meditations

Archangels 101 (abridged audio book)

Solomon's Angels (audio book)

Fairies 101 (abridged audio book)

Angel Medicine (available as both 1- and 2-CD sets)

Angels among Us (with Michael Toms)

Messages from Your Angels (abridged audio book)

Past-Life Regression with the Angels

Divine Prescriptions

The Romance Angels

Connecting with Your Angels

Manifesting with the Angels

Karma Releasing

Healing Your Appetite, Healing Your Life

Healing with the Angels

Divine Guidance

Chakra Clearing

DVD Program

How to Give an Angel Card Reading

Oracle Cards (divination cards and guidebook)

Fairy Tarot Cards (with Radleigh Valentine; available December 2015)

Angel Answers Oracle Cards (with Radleigh Valentine)

Guardian Angel Tarot Cards (with Radleigh Valentine)

Past Life Oracle Cards (with Brian Weiss, M.D.)

Cherub Angel Cards for Children

LIVING
PAIN-FREE

Natural and Spiritual Solutions
to Eliminate Physical Pain

Doreen Virtue
and
Robert Reeves, N.D.

HAY HOUSE, INC.
Carlsbad, California • New York City
London • Sydney • Johannesburg
Vancouver • Hong Kong • New Delhi

Published and distributed in the United States by: Hay House, Inc.: www.hayhouse .com® • *Published and distributed in Australia by:* Hay House Australia Pty. Ltd.: www.hayhouse.com.au • *Published and distributed in the United Kingdom by:* Hay House UK, Ltd.: www.hayhouse.co.uk • *Published and distributed in the Republic of South Africa by:* Hay House SA (Pty), Ltd.: www.hayhouse.co.za • *Distributed in Canada by:* Raincoast Books: www.raincoast.com • *Published in India by:* Hay House Publishers India: www.hayhouse.co.in

Cover design: Amy Rose Grigoriou
Interior design: Nick C. Welch

Library of Congress Cataloging-in-Publication Data

Virtue, Doreen, date, author.
 Living pain-free : natural and spiritual solutions to eliminate physical pain / Doreen Virtue, Robert Reeves. -- 1st edition.
   pages cm
 Includes bibliographical references.
 ISBN 978-1-4019-4411-7 (hardback)
 1. Chronic pain--Alternative treatment. 2. Mental healing. 3. Spiritual healing. 4. Mind and body--Health aspects. I. Reeves, Robert (Naturopath) II. Title.
 RB127.V56 2014
 616'.0472--dc23

                            2014018364

Hardcover ISBN: 978-1-4019-4411-7

10 9 8 7 6 5 4 3 2 1
1st edition, November 2014

Printed in the United States of America

*To those willing
to make the change
from pain to pain-free!*

CONTENTS

INTRODUCTION

You *Can* Live Pain-Free!

Beneath your pain, there is a fully functioning, healthy, comfortable body. Our goal with this book is to help you allow that reality to shine through. To that end, we offer our insights into the causes of pain, as well as suggestions regarding numerous natural prescriptions and spiritual solutions to heal it. We recommend herbal remedies because plants are God's medicine, found in nature and used for centuries by intuitive indigenous healers.

Within these pages, we also mention the concept of the ego, which is an underlying cause of pain. In a spiritual sense, the ego is unlike the word *egotistical,* so just erase those associations for a moment. Instead, think of the expression "an angel on one shoulder and a devil on the other." There are two voices within each of us: one that uplifts us (the angels), and one that attracts fear (the ego). The ego voice says, *You're not good enough, You'll never be well, You should give up,* and *Nobody loves you.* However, these are complete and utter lies! Your angels love you more than you know, and their only desire is to watch you succeed.

The important thing to remember is how to tell the difference between what your ego is saying and what the angels are saying. If you receive a message through thoughts, visions, feelings, or words that is uplifting and positive, you can be assured that it's coming from your angels. If a message makes you feel low or self-conscious, or convinces you not to take the next step, it's likely from your ego.

Everybody has angels; they are healing allies that surround and support you at every moment. You don't need to be religious or saintly—*everyone* has guardian angels around them at all times. It doesn't even matter whether you believe in angels, because they are part of our physiology. They are as vital and natural as our lungs, brain, or heart.

Your angels are with you right now, hoping to infuse your body with the comfort that it needs. You might be wondering, *Then why haven't they already healed me?* It is important to know that angels are bound by the Law of Free Will. This Universal Law states that neither they nor God can intervene in your life without your express permission. You must first ask for help; then miracles can occur. When you speak from your heart, your loving angels will hear every word.

᠊᠊᠊ ᠊᠊᠊ ᠊᠊᠊ ᠊᠊᠊

In the following chapters, we offer a deeper understanding of what pain is, its origins, the role it plays in your body, and how it affects and is affected by your emotions, including stress. We provide suggestions for not only treating your symptoms but also creating true wellness through nutrition, exercise, herbs and supplements, detoxing, and honoring your sensitivity. There is a simple reference guide at the end of this book that lists some of the most common locations for pain in the body; its possible energetic causes; and specific healing recommendations, including therapies, supplements, prayers, and affirmations. You may either read this book straight through or allow your intuition to guide your journey, choosing whichever topics are most relevant for you at a particular time.

Remember that with any health issue, it's best to also seek proper medical advice. If you've had chronic, undiagnosed pain, make an appointment to see a qualified health professional; a diagnosis may help you in your quest for comfort. Consult a health-care professional before altering medications or introducing new things into your routine, such as exercise or nutritional supplements. Particular remedies will not be appropriate for everyone, so if you have pre-existing conditions or are currently on a treatment regimen, seek advice to be certain that what you're guided to take will not interact with your medication or aggravate your symptoms.

We must use the safest approaches to our health and, above all, do no harm. Please be sensible and informed as you explore the many approaches to alleviating pain.

Enjoy your journey to a completely comfortable and pain-free life.

— Doreen and Robert

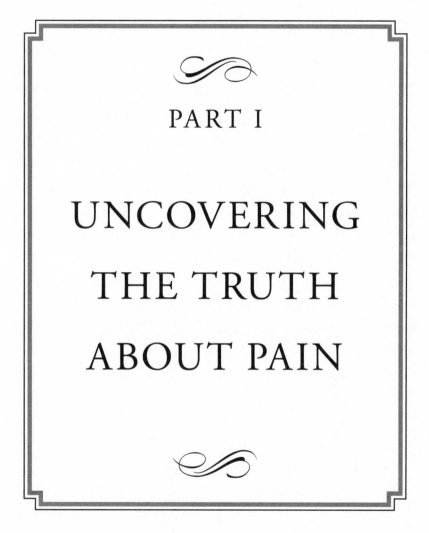

PART I

UNCOVERING THE TRUTH ABOUT PAIN

CHAPTER ONE

THE ORIGINS OF PAIN

If you let it, pain can ruin your life.

Now, read that sentence again . . . the key words are *if you let it.*

Your future is in your hands. Don't give up the fight just yet. In this book you will find numerous ways to heal from physical ailments. The pain that might have once held you back is quivering in its boots. It knows that here you will gain the tools necessary to change your life. You can overcome the obstacle of pain and throw off the shackles that were binding you.

You might have lost your focus while trying to read this book, or become distracted when you tried to address your discomfort, because your ego is terrified by the possibility of relief. Your ego distracts you, because if you were healed, you would be in the perfect place to complete your life purpose. Suffering limits your feelings of joy, which then causes your purpose in life to elude you. However, as soon as the cloud of pain is lifted, the road ahead is crystal clear. This allows you to easily see your true calling.

Every thought you have is helping to shape your reality and your experiences. So by focusing their thoughts around pain, some people attract others who also suffer. Notice who is in your circle of friends. Do you have high-energy, uplifting people in your life? Or are you surrounded only by others who are struggling, limited, and dark in their outlook? The point of this exercise isn't to judge or criticize ourselves, but rather to identify aspects we might like to change. Just as you had the power to attract these people, you have the power to attract happy, healthy friends, too.

The limitation of pain convinces you that you're trapped. It tells you that progress will be difficult and that you can't move forward. If you listen to that voice, then you will lose inspiration, motivation, and creativity—three things that are essential for getting out and making a difference in the world.

You're here to do much more than merely exist. It is natural to contemplate why you are here at this time. The reason is because your soul carries with it Divine wisdom that's desperately needed on Earth right now. On some level you know this statement to be true. Imagine what your life would be like if you felt inspired every moment. Imagine what it would look like if you followed through on all of your heart's desires. This is what living pain-free is like.

So now let's remove the old energy of pain and usher in your incredible future!

What Is Pain?

Pain is a sign that something is unbalanced in your body. Taking anti-inflammatories and analgesic medications only masks the discomfort, without actually addressing the cause. Rather than covering up the messages of your body, try to decipher what it's saying.

The true cause of your hurt may be physical, emotional, or energetic. Regardless of what the reason may be, do not judge yourself or your experiences—doing so would only add to your suffering. Look at your situation objectively. Ask yourself: *When did the pain begin? What else was going on during that time in my life? Were there other stressors or traumas?* You may be surprised to find that your body is reflecting something that is or was occurring in your life.

When new patients come to see me (Robert) in my naturopathic practice, they may be hoping that I will prescribe something to ease their pain. While I always offer support in some fashion, it is not necessarily in the way they expect. There is no point in taking something to mask your symptoms, because the underlying issue is still there. As soon as you stop the medication, your troubles will return. This is why, whenever I meet people in my practice for the first time, we always sit and talk about what else is or was happening in their lives.

One patient realized that her suffering began the same time her relationship with her husband got rocky. Anytime she and her partner argued, her discomfort increased. Until that point, she had never connected the dots. Her body was using physical pain to mask her emotional pain so that she wouldn't have to face her feelings! Not surprisingly she had a lot of old emotions stored up and hidden away. As she became comfortable releasing them, her pain began to lessen until it completely left her body, mind, and spirit. Now would taking painkillers have solved a problem like that? Not likely!

Once you understand where your pain originates, you must look at its severity and frequency. Ask yourself:

- *When does the discomfort become worse?*
- *What else is happening at those times—am I more stressed?*
- *Did I just spend time with someone, or eat or drink something?*
- *When does the pain ease, and when do I feel at my best?*
- *What activities, emotions, or relationships am I experiencing at these times?*

The answers to these questions contain vital clues to your path to wellness. By recognizing the actions that bring you comfort, you can commit yourself to doing them more frequently. On the other hand, when you realize what increases your suffering, you can choose to separate yourself from those situations.

The Illusion of Pain

In spiritual truth your body is already healed. Your soul carries with it all the information you need to venture down the path to a comfortable, happy, loving life. It is when you listen to the fear-based thoughts of your ego that you waver from this path and experience pain as a result.

We have compassion for the very real suffering that you are experiencing. However, you must remember that the way God has created you is Divinely perfect. God, being pure love, would not have created pain. Your discomfort is not a spiritual test, but a product of the ego, which is the opposite of God. To buy into it is to give energy to something that's not from our Creator.

Look past the illusion of suffering and instead view your body for what it is in truth. Pain is using your body for its home; serve it an eviction notice and tell it that it's no longer welcome in your sacred temple. Remove the blocks that are dimming your light. Such obstructions on your path to pure health may include chemicals and toxins in foods and beverages, negative thought patterns, low-energy environments, poor diet, lack of exercise, and dis-ease.

Note that we distinguish *dis-ease* from disease. When you say "I have a disease," it is a label that continually affirms poor health. On the other hand, a state of dis-ease is simply saying that you aren't in your best condition in this moment and that you need to restore a sense of balance.

It is important to avoid saying things like "*my* sore back . . ." "*my* pain . . ." and "everything always hurts." With phrasing such as this, you claim ownership of the condition—do you really want it to be *your* pain? When you release suffering from your vocabulary, you can also choose to exchange it for love, health, and peace. The universe is always listening to you and attracting to you what you give out, and negative statements like these send your energy out to perpetuate your current state.

To make things easier, imagine that you have a genie with you at every moment, listening to every thought and every feeling that you have. It wants to grant your wishes, and it thinks that you want more of whatever it is that you focus on. Help the genie by always "asking" for what you want, rather than keeping your attention on what you don't.

Put your energy to its best use by affirming the positive. Say things like "My back is flexible and strong," "My body is comfortable," and "I feel better every day as I continue to heal," even if you don't fully believe it at the time you say it. As long as you're willing to have patience with the process, such statements will help bring your attention to, and eventually bring about, the positive condition that you are affirming.

During our personal meditations, we asked the angels how willing someone needed to be in order to heal from discomfort. On a scale ranging from 0 to 10, with 10 being the most willing, the angels said they only needed a 1. Even the slightest hint of willingness is enough for the angels to create positive changes in your life. So despite what the rational mind may be saying, the only thing you have to lose is pain.

Different Types of Pain

There are generally three different areas of physical pain that we can experience: *muscle, nerve,* and *bone.*

— **Muscle** aches are the most common, as well as the most generalized. It can often be difficult to distinguish the exact area that hurts the most. You might have a sore neck or back, but there isn't one specific spot you can really pinpoint. Instead, a whole area may feel affected, like a band across your back, or the pain may spread. An ache tends to occur when a muscle is tense, which makes blood flow more difficult. As the muscle lacks blood, it begins to send the signal of pain.

— **Nerves** are responsible for all movements that occur in your body. The brain sends signals along them to your muscles so that you can move appropriately. Occasionally a nerve becomes trapped between tense muscles; then, as you move, it gets pinched, which triggers sharp, sudden, and often severe pain—it can even take your breath away!

The signal can run through the entire length of a pinched nerve. Sciatica, which affects the nerve that extends from the lower back and down each leg, is one of the most common examples. So while you may have discomfort running down your leg, for instance, the actual impingement may be in your lower back. With nerve pain, the specific path can usually be pinpointed, and you can show a health practitioner exactly where the discomfort starts and where it extends.

— **Bone** pain is a deep pain. It doesn't change with muscle movements. It should always be taken seriously, as it may indicate fracture, infection, or cancer. Please have bone pain investigated by a qualified medical professional.

Common Causes of Pain

It is necessary to acknowledge the source of your pain in order to effectively heal it. Beware of treatments that just address symptoms superficially, without getting to the root of things. Following those methods will necessitate repeating the process again and again, because the real repair work has not been done. Know that with true healing, once the issue is resolved, the pain leaves your body and cannot return.

That being said, it may take some time for you to achieve true well-being. Don't feel limited to any particular remedy; you may work with natural as well as conventional methods, as you feel guided to do so. Some therapists suggest that for every year you've had an issue, it will take one month to treat it. So according to this theory, if you've had back pain for five years, it may take up to five months to clear it fully. The more open and willing you are to let go of your suffering, the faster it can leave. You'll attain as much healing as you're willing to receive.

The following are the most common reasons why you may be in pain.

Wear and Tear

Over time, things can simply wear out. This is true for all objects, including your body and its joints. If you were highly active in your youth or played rough sports like football, rugby, motocross, or skiing, your joints may have taken quite a beating. This can lead to arthritis and stiffness later in life. Ingesting nourishing oils, such as flaxseed, will help keep those joints well lubricated.

You don't have to focus on the negative in the situation here. If you played sports, you likely enjoyed them a great deal. Bring your attention to the happiness that these activities gave you, rather than what the future may or may not hold. You can take good care of yourself now, and set yourself up for a long and comfortable life.

Aging

Age is a natural progression of life. Many people say that it is simply fact that as we get older, we experience more pain.

Let's examine that belief for a moment. What comes first: the discomfort or the self-fulfilling prophecy? Perhaps what creates the pain is the constant affirmation that it is inevitable. This is a great insight—if your brain has the ability to create a situation, then it also holds the key to its alleviation! If your mind can create it, your mind can change it. Focus on being a youthful spirit, and your body will follow suit.

Weight

Your body is created with a Divine balance, a delicate structure that has a built-in optimal weight. If you carry extra pounds, it puts strain on your muscles and joints. It makes your heart work harder in order to push blood around a larger body. Over time, your spine can start to compress as your core muscles lose strength. If you're overweight, losing some weight can drastically decrease your discomfort. Every extra pound that you carry is an extra pound of pain your body must manage.

There are many reasons a person might be overweight, including poor diet, stress, or hormonal imbalance:

— *Diet:* You can do far more damage to your body with the food you consume than can be counteracted by any amount of exercise. You can work out for over an hour, then undo all that good work in a matter of minutes! High-calorie, low-nutrient foods are easily accessible, and often contain artificial preservatives and sweeteners that actually inhibit weight loss. Also, be wary of any food touted as "diet" or sugar-free, because many of these items contain additives that have been linked to cancers and other health complaints. When you remove them from your life, you will immediately notice improvement in your comfort level.

— *Stress:* When you are under stress, it triggers your body to release the hormone cortisol. This hormone increases your appetite and also attracts fluid and bulks you up. Its main role is to help your body cope with whatever burden you are under. It is wonderfully useful in small doses. However, if you experience long-term stress, then you may have too much cortisol floating around in your system.

— *Hormones:* If your hormones are unbalanced, then you may become fatigued and lethargic. You might lose motivation to do the activities that once brought you joy. You know the things that can help you, but instead you procrastinate and delay your getting better. Fluctuating hormone levels may cause you to feel good one day and depressed the next.

If you suspect that your hormones are unbalanced, please get examined by a qualified health-care professional. You may accidentally do more harm than good if you try to create a treatment plan based on a self-diagnosis. Accept support from someone who is trained in what to do.

Food

Dietary factors play a critical role in your health, apart from your weight. Some foods trigger immune responses that can cause you physical discomfort. It is also important to note that your body is happiest in an alkaline state. In this situation, your cells function well and there is not much inflammation. However, some foods are considered more acidic than others, and they disrupt the balance in your body. (We discuss how to maintain an alkaline diet, as well as how to improve your overall nutrition intake, in Chapter 5.)

Lack of Exercise

Your ego might tell you that working out will only make your pain worse, but the truth is that avoiding activity actually *delays* your improvement. Regular exercise helps loosen tight muscles, lubricate your joints, and regulate your metabolism. (In Chapter 7, we'll go over different exercises and ways to start incorporating them into your life.)

If you are sedentary, or if you are sitting for most of the day, your pelvis can start to tilt. As your body tries to adjust for this misalignment, your back is put under more strain. Then, in an effort to ease your aching back, you might avoid too much movement. However, if you had continually done careful stretching and gentle activities, your pelvis could have corrected itself earlier.

If you feel that your height has decreased, it may be because your spine is compressed. If this degradation is due to a reduction in bone density, then there may not be anything you can do about it. But if it was a recent change, you can use regular movement and stretching to readjust your body. A gentle yoga or beginners' Pilates class can have wonderful curative effects. Having a strong and sturdy core will give you a long spine and comfortable back.

Living with Pain

There are now more people than ever living with chronic pain. This is just one of the many reasons we felt guided to write this book. So many people are waking each day to a life of suffering. As we share with you our knowledge, the messages from the angels, and other people's firsthand experiences in this book, know that you can heal through this and live a truly pain-free life.

According to the Australian Bureau of Statistics, there were about 11 million Australians aged 15 years and older who experienced pain within the last four weeks prior to being surveyed. Approximately one in ten Australians reported feeling severe to very severe pain.

Likewise, a report from the Institute of Medicine found that at least 100 million Americans suffer from serious chronic pain every year. Some would consider this number conservative, as it does not take children into account, nor acute pain. The cost of this suffering in lost productivity and medical bills equates to $560 billion to $635 billion per year.

One in five American adults says that pain interrupts their sleep patterns. It is easy to see how challenging it is to go to sleep if you're uncomfortable. By easing your burden, you receive the rest that you need. On a physical level, sleep is your body's time to repair and recharge; without proper rest, you cannot heal fully and completely. On an emotional level, it is essential because it is when you go into your dreamtime, a space where you connect with your angels and your subconscious mind.

Why does it seem that there are so many more people living with chronic pain now than in the past? Along with the increases in population, the proportion of people suffering has also risen. Perhaps it's due to the extra pressure and stress that comes with our modern world. For instance, a common source of worry is that as the years go by, things become more expensive. Perhaps we hold on to the limiting belief that we will continue to earn the same amount as last year, so how would we expect to be able to support ourselves with the added expenses? We must release limitations such as this, and allow the universe to provide for all our earthly needs. It is at this point of surrendering that we are able to receive. Until then, our busy hands are in the way and the angels patiently observe until we give them the space to intervene.

Today so many are put into high-pressure situations. They constantly strive to please others while being asked to meet unrealistic demands. These expectations are not limited to the workplace, either. Society bombards us with images of how we should look, what we need to buy and wear, and where we are meant to be. If we fall for these traps, we succumb to the feelings of failure. Nobody deserves to feel this way! Empower yourself by listening to the inner voice of your angels that encourages and supports you. This process of upliftment will come to you when you're ready. Now is the time!

෬ ෭

CHAPTER TWO

Mind Over Pain

Pain is, essentially, a natural occurrence and meant to be used as a warning sign. For example, if you touched a hot stove, your body would register the sensation of heat and danger, and quickly pull away. Without this instinctive response, you could cause yourself harm. Problems arise, however, when the "pain switch" gets stuck on and never seems to turn off. Chronic discomfort is a sign of an unhappy body.

It is important to understand that living a pain-free life means more than continually popping pills to mask your ailments. Underneath this illusion of suffering is a healthy, comfortable body. For a deeper healing, you must raise your vibration and lift your energy to meet the true vision of yourself. Let's recall what that feels like:

> *Bring your mind back to a time when you felt that there was comfort and ease in every aspect of your life. Perhaps this was during a wonderful vacation that you spent with loved ones. Let go of your worries for now and allow your body to relax. There is no stress, anger, or confrontation in this moment. Feel how your life is balanced, harmonious, and peaceful. Release your expectations; you don't need to tell God how He should heal you. Let events unfold as they will. Trust that God has the*

perfect journey planned for you and that you have always been Divinely protected.

Now let's take a closer look at how pain is triggered and how we can use our minds to overcome it.

The Pathway of Pain

Your body receives messages of discomfort by picking up on reactions occurring in your system, then sending the signal of "pain" to the brain. First, nerve receptors get information and put out an electrical impulse with the message. The impulse travels through nerves, to the spinal cord, then up to your brain. Your thalamus sends it to different parts of your brain to interpret the signal and decides what area should respond first. The result will be a physical response, a thought process, or an emotional reaction.

The brain influences your perception of pain. I (Robert) lose all signs of bravery when shown a needle. If I require a blood test, I can't bear the thought of watching it—syringes, needles, and blood are not a good combination for me. So I always, without exception, look away, and most of the time I feel very little during the procedure. I did notice, though, that even after a test is complete, I could still make the area hurt. If I look at the bandage and think about what happened, I will instantly feel a sharp, pricking sensation. However, as soon as I look away, the feeling eases.

When I meditated on this intriguing phenomenon, my inner guidance told me that the brain could both cause *and* remove pain. If you focus your attention on something that you enjoy, the feeling of suffering disappears. It leaves your body, mind, and aura because it cannot exist within a happy soul. Consider a headache; chances are, if you were distracted or engrossed in a friend's story, the discomfort would be completely gone. If the friend then asked about your headache, you would notice the pain reappearing.

The gate control theory of pain suggests that the mind has the capability to shut down messages signaling that the body has been hurt. Basically, the brain will be either open or closed to receiving pain. Think of athletes playing sports who don't realize until after the game that they are injured. This is because their brains were too preoccupied with other activities to acknowledge the discomfort.

There are several factors that can alter your pain pathway, including age, gender, cultural background, psychological health, upbringing, and your expectation of pain. Let's examine that last factor more closely.

The Expectation of Pain

Pain has the ability to consume your life . . . but only if you allow it. Remember that you are on a journey, and you choose what direction you want to move every day. This is why it is important, as you awake, to express gratitude for the many blessings that have been bestowed upon you. If you instead rise each morning with your mind turned toward what hurts in your life, the universe delivers according to your expectation.

Deep down, you know you don't want this suffering. Your subconscious mind also knows that focusing on it only makes it worse. So think instead about the love in your life and the things that bring you happiness. There are a couple of simple techniques we suggest you try in order to shift your focus.

— Begin by writing down a list of activities that fill you with joy. Take out your journal or a notepad and jot down the many things in your life that you have cause to feel grateful for. Instantly your mood will lift, and your circumstances will seem improved. Remember that pain is merely an illusion that the ego tries to convince you of. Rather than paying attention to it, listen to your angels, who will show you ways of expressing your true health.

— For the second method, you need to get a special box. At the end of each day, cut up a piece of paper and write down a blessing you experienced on each tiny slip. Describe what made you feel good, happy interactions you shared with others, and the miracles you saw. Then place these notes inside the box. Whenever you feel low or distracted by pain, you can take out one of these slips to read. You'll quickly feel the beauty of your own words and remember the pure enjoyment you've experienced in the gift that is your life. It is a reminder that all suffering is temporary; there is always the opportunity to reconnect with peace.

෧෮

Just because a belief was true for you once in the past, it does not mean that it must be true for you now. While certain activities may have caused you discomfort at one time, holding on to those memories causes your body to expect to hurt again in those circumstances each time thereafter. This is why it is important to also remember the joy that those same events brought to you.

For example, perhaps the prospect of a long car ride brings back memories of being cramped and achy—but can you remember what you did at your destination? Did you take a long trip to the city and engage in joyful activities that made you smile? If you connect with the positive instead of the negative energy, you'll find your relationship with travel beginning to change.

You can use this method for any activity. Just because you awoke with pain this morning, it doesn't need to be true tomorrow. Don't allow your ego to trick you into believing otherwise; push the "delete" button on all those old associations. We'll keep the love and embrace the joy, but erase the pain.

Your thoughts are like fish swimming down the current of a stream. They continue with the momentum of their journey. If you wake in the morning and expect to feel discomfort, you can redirect the flow from your stream of thoughts to focus upon peace and ease. However, if you continue to stay with negative thoughts surrounding pain, it's like trying to change the course of a river as it rushes down a mountain. It's far easier to alter in the beginning compared to when the momentum has picked up speed.

Create a new expectation of comfort and ease: Tomorrow you will wake completely comfortable and rested. The car trip to the city will be smooth and pain-free. Expect the best situation to occur . . . and it will.

Take Time to Shine

When life gets busy, it can be easy to allow your hobbies and other interests to slip away—but that is precisely when you most need them! Without connecting to your passion, you begin to feel depleted and exhausted. All joy leaves you, your light is dimmed, and soon enough, pain arrives.

You must remember that you are a beautiful example of God's manifested love. When you allow your Divine light to shine, you let others know that there's hope. You can inspire people to join you on a happy, healing path. Indeed, the angels are asking you *right now* to let your light shine; it is essential to your well-being! When you simply take time to enjoy life, your body responds with health, and you feel brighter and happier.

Even if you are incredibly busy, schedule time for your hobbies and for play. No one wants to live in a reality where you have to work every waking minute. Sure, your work can be rewarding and fun, but it also helps provide the tools necessary for your enjoyment. Yet so many have forgotten the second phase of working. They make the money but forget to spend it on fun and comfort.

Highly successful people keep this principle in mind. They enjoy what they do and embrace joy in their lives. They find exciting ways to fulfill their commitments, keeping their energy and motivation high.

If you don't reward yourself, you begin to resent your job, and this can be a further obstacle to your healing. If you aren't finding pleasure in what you do, then change it. Begin by using affirmations to create a reality that you *will* enjoy. Affirmations are positive statements in the present tense that you repeat to yourself in order to manifest a desired outcome.

To affirm your desires and dreams, try saying:

- "My life fulfills me in all ways."

- "Each moment brings me greater joy."

- "I am open to receiving all good; this allows me to give to others more freely."

- "My career is deeply fulfilling and rewarding."
- "Every day is a new opportunity to experience love."

Repeating affirmations to yourself during your daily activities will help bring your focus back to your goals. Initially it may feel like you are lying to yourself. Your ego resists these uplifting words in favor of the negative thoughts it's familiar with. With continual repetition, your subconscious begins to believe your affirmations; then you are in a position to start taking steps to *make* the statements true.

If you spend the majority of your day at a job, you need to enjoy it. By loving what you do, you no longer feel like you're working. Instead, you're getting paid to play and have fun. This approach brings you the perspective you need on your path toward comfort and joy.

Meditations for Easing Your Pain

Since your brain has the power to bring sensations into reality, it can also remove them for good. Use this to your advantage by training your mind in meditation or guided imagery. Taking your attention away from pain will bring you the greatest joy of all. The following are a few of our favorites that you might like to try.

Therapeutic Ocean

Visualize yourself walking along a beautiful beach at sunset or sunrise. Affirm that the temperature is perfect. There is just enough sea breeze, and your feet enjoy the gentle caress of the sand and waves. Feel the ocean taking away all of your concerns and washing them off. You do not need to hold on to these old emotions, as they are not doing you or anyone else any favors. Take time to breathe deeply and enjoy this magical experience.

Healing Rain Forest

See yourself seated in the middle of a rain forest. Take time to notice the many shades of green that surround you. Green is the color of healing, which you welcome into your body. You will likely experience tingling sensations as the emerald energy enters your being.

With you in the rain forest is Archangel Raphael. He will clear away any obstacles to your peace and well-being. Listen to the sounds of nature—the trees and birds—and the sweet song of serenity.

Higher Perspective

Take your mind to the top of a mountain. From here you're able to gain new perspectives. Sit down on a purple rug and observe the beauty below you. Understand that when you rise, you have the decision of where you want to go. Do you want to go back to the way you were before—or do you want to accept greater health, well-being, and love?

You may feel a strong presence with you. This is Archangel Michael, who is here to help clear away fear and negative energies from your life. He will protect you and keep you safe from all harm. He understands that you've had difficulties in the past, but wishes to illuminate the path to your true healing. Genuine relief can only come from inside you. It isn't something that you receive from others. It's something that shines within you from the moment you were born.

Your true state of Divine health is already beaming brightly. Ask God and the angels to clear away the darkness so that your light can once again be revealed. As you do so, others will be inspired by your journey and join you on the path of joy. This is the magic of healing with the angels; they not only focus upon your needs, but send their energy outward to create won-drous experiences everywhere you go.

You are a shining example of God's love. You deserve abso-lute health and comfort. Spend time in this meditation to gain the most healing you can.

❧

When you're in any of these meditative states, you can always ask your angels for additional information and support. Simply think the phrase: *Angels, what else do you want me to know right now? What changes would you like to see me make?*

Then listen with all of your body. Pay attention to any thoughts, feelings, visions, or sounds. Please also realize that there is no such thing as a coincidence; everything is perfectly orches-trated for you to notice along your path. Rather than dismissing something, look harder—perhaps you will recognize it as the an-swer to your prayers.

For example, I (Doreen) received a letter from Paula Kucner Taipa from Poland. She said she enjoyed listening to my weekly show on Hay House Radio. One day, Paula had a terrible headache and a toothache. During the show that week, I guided the listeners through a healing meditation with the angels. Paula felt the pain lift out of her body—it completely dissipated! She gratefully gave the situation over to God and enjoyed the benefits of meditation. You can, too!

❧ ❧

CHAPTER THREE

A Look at Stress and Inflammation

It is easy to allow pain to take center stage in your life. You might think that the stress you are under is a secondary issue; perhaps you even blame your physical discomfort for creating the emotional strain to begin with. While this may be partly true, it is important to acknowledge the impact your emotions can have on your wonderful body.

Stress is one of the biggest obstacles to well-being. If you continue to listen to the voice of fear, then you let yourself fall into a cycle of pain. When you recognize that worrying does no good, you can more easily let your cares go. By taking a multifaceted approach to your wellness, you are more likely to achieve better, and permanent, results.

Allow your angels to support you; choose to pray for a better situation rather than continuing with unproductive stress. You will be Divinely helped on your healing path if you open the doors for Heaven to ease your burdens. However, until you grant permission, you walk down the path unaided. Of course, your angels and God are with you always, but they can't interfere with your freewill choices.

Keeping in mind this spiritual truth, it becomes clear that stress is something we must not let into our lives. The angels share with us that stress is simply:

Some

Time

Requiring

Energy

Starving

Spirituality

By that definition, the energy expended in stress does no good, only creating more strain. It blocks your spiritual communication and tricks you into wasting useful time. Choose to replace it with the beneficial energy of joy, peace, and healing.

The angels want you to think of activities that you love. Ask yourself the question: *When did I last spend time doing any of those things?* If it was longer than last week, you need to adjust your priorities in order to help yourself be stress-free as well as pain-free. Take time each week to do what makes you feel good. Make an appointment with yourself, and promise that you'll do what you love. Don't allow money issues to be an excuse; you don't need to have regular spa appointments or expensive massages. There are many simple activities you can turn to instead. For example, you might enjoy a relaxing bath at home, quiet time to read, or a peaceful walk in nature. Whatever it is that brings you joy will be worth it.

The angels will provide, so that you have everything you need to be happy. If regular massages really would bring you peace, then pray for it. You needn't feel guilty about this or think that you're wasting God's time. Heaven knows that the more comfortable and happy you are, the more likely it is that you will listen to your inner guidance, complete your purpose, and make a real difference in your own life as well as the lives of others. The angels simply want you to be happy, so your asking for these things isn't insulting to them. They know that it's not the material objects that are important, but the love that is exchanged. Any activity in which you feel nurtured and loved will be worth the angelic investment.

To further illustrate our point, remember the safety demonstrations on an airplane. Before each flight, the attendants remind you that, in case of emergency, you must put the oxygen mask on yourself before you help others. This is because *you* first need the air to breathe; you must attend to your own needs before you can be of service to anyone else. If you ignore this important self-care principle, then you'd likely lose consciousness and be unable to assist anyone—including yourself!

The angels remind us that everyday life abides by the same rules. You must take a moment to care for your needs before worrying yourself with other people's issues. Remember to check in and see where the stress you feel is coming from. Is a situation in your own life creating it, or is it coming from another person? If it's coming from other people's energy, then you can easily clear it by calling upon Archangel Michael and engaging in regular shielding. Imagine a barrier of energy surrounding you, protecting you from others' negativity and outside influences. You can invoke or strengthen your shield whenever you feel you need it. (Chapter 11 offers more information on shielding.) If you think that *you* are the source of your stress, pray for guidance. Ask God and your guardian angels to share with you new ways in which to proceed.

The Effects of Chronic Stress on Your Body

If we think back to only a few decades ago, modern medicine didn't even consider stress a health concern. Today it's commonly recognized as the root of a number of conditions. Long-term stress increases the levels of the hormone cortisol in your body, which in turn increases inflammation and promotes the development and progression of many diseases. It triggers a multitude of unfortunate bodily responses and leaves you feeling frazzled.

As a visual aid, imagine an electrical cable. Now picture what would happen if you took off the coating and pulled all the wires apart. This is similar to what stress does to your nervous system.

It frays everything so your body's messages are harder to process. It takes you a longer time to adjust to change, and your natural healing pathways are blocked.

It is important to ensure that you have an outlet to release any mental or emotional strain you are under. The angels say that, like a closet, we have a limited number of "shelves," and right now some of yours may be filled with stress energy and old emotions. Even if you tried to welcome new love, healing, or positive energy into your life, it would have nowhere to go. This is why it is so necessary to clear away some of the clutter from those shelves—by making new room, you allow the healing to enter.

Healthy ways to let go of stress include meditation, tai chi, and prayer. Exercise is also a wonderful relief because it triggers your body to produce a rush of endorphins, your feel-good hormones. Try to spend some time outdoors to enjoy the sunshine. As the golden rays touch your skin, be willing to let go of all that no longer serves you. Allow the warmth from the heavenly sun to purify your heart, mind, and soul.

Writing letters is another good way to release your emotions. To start, simply sit at your computer and type a letter that express-es your feelings—then close the program without saving your work. Nobody needs to reads your thoughts, but it is essential that you get them out of your energy field. Once those old things have been cleared, there's space for healing energy and love to reside.

The Role of Inflammation

Psychological stress increases your levels of cortisol and leads to chronic inflammation in your body. It's important to note that inflammation can be the biggest helper and yet also the biggest hindrance to healing. It is a signal to the body to begin repair work in the isolated area. Helpful cells are sent to the affected site to aid recovery. These serve to keep nasty invaders at bay, such as bacteria and viruses, and they protect the area from further damage.

However, when inflammation becomes an ongoing condition, it promotes the development and progression of many ailments.

Chronic inflammation often does not have characteristic symptoms you can see with the naked eye, such as redness. Yet fluid buildup and swelling may be apparent, perpetuating the inflammation. This extra pressure can cause more pain and prevent the body from healing. Long-term inflammation also leads to the production of damaging free radicals, which age your cells prematurely and contribute to a whole host of health conditions, including cardiovascular disease and cancer.

There are certain cases in which your immune system mistakenly triggers inflammatory responses. Such conditions include asthma, where your airways (the tiny tubes that transport air to your lungs) become swollen and narrowed, inhibiting breathing. High blood pressure can be affected by inflammation in the kidneys. Abdominal cramps and diarrhea may be caused by an inflamed colon. If you experience any of these conditions, reducing your levels of stress will lead to less overall inflammation in your body, which may ease or eliminate flare-ups.

Many people believe that they should remain sedentary in order to let themselves heal—however, this actually causes inflammation to increase. It will sit in your body until you clear it. This is why it is essential to include regular exercise as part of your routine. Start with gentle walking. Then, as your fitness builds, you can incorporate more strenuous workouts. You can refer to Chapter 7 for suggestions on how to build your exercise regimen.

One important way to reduce chronic inflammation is to consume enough omega-3 oils. Make sure you supplement with flaxseed oil, which helps properly lubricate your joints and release your muscles. We discuss omega-3s in the next chapter, along with other supplements and herbs with pain-relieving properties.

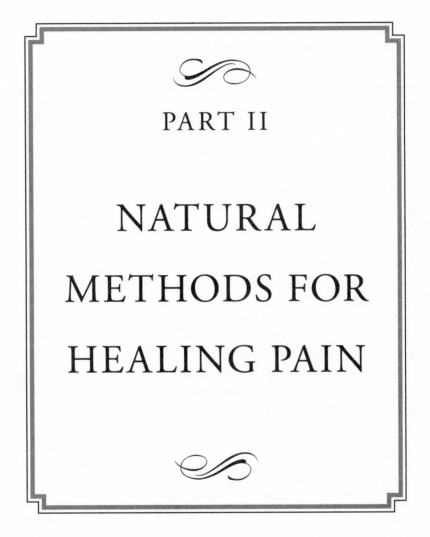

PART II

NATURAL METHODS FOR HEALING PAIN

CHAPTER FOUR

Pain-Relieving
Herbal Medicines
and Supplements

Herbal medicines are a wonderful way to connect with the energy of the earth, and your body responds to them beautifully. There's no resistance. There's no heavy manipulation of your delicate system. Instead, the herbs support your body to create a state of wellness.

It is interesting that many pharmaceutical drugs have plant-based origins or are simply modified forms of compounds derived from plants. You may ask yourself, "Why don't we just use the natural versions instead of trying to copy what God perfected?" Well, the simple answer is that there's no money to be made that way—you cannot patent something that naturally exists. Pharmaceutical companies re-create these compounds in a laboratory, then hope that the body will respond to the manufactured compound the same way it does to the natural substance. They also tend to isolate or focus on one particular chemical. On the other hand, natural remedies acknowledge the wonderful team of plant-based compounds that work in symphony to create a healing effect.

We do believe there's a place for both modern medicine and traditional therapies. If, God forbid, we experienced a broken leg or dislocated shoulder, we would certainly consider pharmaceutical treatment as a valid option. That said, we feel that spiritual and natural remedies provide the most benefits in addressing chronic pain, whether constant or recurring.

Of course, pain medications serve a purpose and can help in acute, severe situations. However many people become dependent on them and experience a range of terrible side effects. Stomach upsets and digestive discomfort are quite common; if you are sensitive, then harsh, chemical-based remedies will only cause you greater misery. Focus instead on natural alternatives that your body can easily tolerate and appropriately use. (In the Appendix, you'll find natural "prescriptions" to ease pain in specific areas of the body.)

The Risk of Pharmaceuticals

One of the most frightening and, unfortunately, all-too-common results of the use of pharmaceutical medication is overdose. Statistics from the Centers for Disease Control (CDC) in the United States reveal that in 2009, there were 475,000 visits to the emergency room by people who had misused or abused pain medication. In 2008, more than 30,000 people died from an overdose of prescription drugs, and of these, pain medications were involved in 14,800 deaths—more than the number of deaths involving heroin and cocaine *combined*. Since 1990, the number of drug-related deaths in the U.S. has more than tripled; in this same time period, the number of prescriptions for pain medication has also increased by 300 percent. I (Doreen) lost a dear friend who passed away at age 55 from a heart attack triggered by taking too many prescription pain pills.

When people take a painkiller, the chemicals latch onto receptor sites in the brain, which causes the pain to go away. Often, they also feel a mild state of euphoria, and it is not uncommon to become addicted to that comfortable feeling. The irrational mind is seduced into taking more pills to achieve an even greater blissful state.

It is important to know that pain medication can act as a sedative. If a high enough dosage is taken, breathing can slow down so much that it stops. It's a dangerous practice for addicted users, who try to strike a balance between dosages that are high enough to take away withdrawal symptoms and give them the euphoria they crave, yet low enough not to jeopardize their lives. The sheer number of deaths that occur each year is a clear sign that this practice is extremely risky and cannot be maintained for long.

A terrifying number of people are using painkillers recreationally. In 2010, the CDC reported that more than 12 million Americans used pain medications for the feeling they got when they took them rather than for management of their symptoms. This is evidence of painkillers' highly addictive nature and the risk they pose for sensitive people. If you are reading this book, you are most likely a sensitive person. You're seeking answers to questions that most others have yet to explore. We're not here to shame modern medicine or steer you away from it. Instead we want you to know the facts. An educated person is better at making a wise decision for his or her health and future.

Herbal Remedies

An alternative to prescription painkillers, herbal medicines can come in tablets, capsules, tinctures, or extracts. As long as the quality of the herb is the same, the form in which you ingest it shouldn't make a difference. However, liquid forms require less work from your system because they are already broken down and ready to be absorbed. Tablets, in contrast, need to be digested before the precious medicines can be utilized by your body.

When purchasing herbal remedies, look first for organic or biodynamic products. This usually means the plants have been grown without the use of chemicals and pesticides, and with farming practices that aren't harmful to the environment. Wild-crafted herbs are also very potent. These are herbs that have been picked in their natural environment. Finally, there are conventionally or trade-grown herbs, which have been treated with harsh fertilizers, chemicals, and pesticides. Be careful; when you ingest these, you may also be putting harmful toxins into your body.

Not every company puts information about how their herbs are grown on their labels, but you can certainly ask for it. Don't become complacent about what you're putting into your body. Give yourself the best chance of recovery by avoiding toxins and poor-quality products. If you are sensitive to alcohol for whatever reason, be sure to check whether your liquid herbs are suspended in alcohol. There are plenty of herbs in nonalcoholic suspensions.

Healing Prayer Over Herbs

Before taking your herbs, pay your respects to the plant for its act of service. Take a few moments to infuse your medicine with love and gratitude. This will raise its vibration and increase its effectiveness.

Either place the herb in your hands, or hold your hands just above it. Connect to its energy by breathing deeply. As you relax through this conscious breath, your aura expands. Let your energy mingle with that of the herb. You'll feel a slight pressure, tingling, or warmth in your hands.

Next, call upon the healing energy of Archangel Raphael by saying:

"Dear God and Archangel Raphael, please infuse this healing herb with your energy. I thank this herb for its act of service. I ask this sacred plant, which you created, to heal my physical body, my emotions, and my energy. Please bring me all that I need at this time."

Visualize the herbal medicine glowing with a very bright white light. Know that this will integrate with your body easily and effortlessly. Next, say:

"Angels, I ask you to awaken the spirit of this herb for healing. May your gift of service be well received. Thank you."

Now, allow the herb to do its healing work.

Choose Herbs and Supplements Intuitively

Follow your intuition when choosing herbal medicines. If you get a gut feeling to try a certain herb, trust it—the results could be life changing. (Of course, if you are under medical care, check with a professional to ensure safety in terms of interactions with your current medications.)

Elena Vasilis discovered the healing power of herbs when she was in her early 20s. She suffered from constant digestive pain, nausea, and discomfort. Her doctor would prescribe antibiotics, but the symptoms never went away. After a couple of years, a doctor arranged an endoscopy and discovered that Elena had acid reflux disease. She was prescribed stomach tablets, but she continued to experience discomfort. She prayed for a miracle from God and Archangel Raphael.

Then Elena decided to take action and began taking better care of herself. She started eating more fruits and vegetables and drinking more water. She also decided to remove gluten and dairy from her diet, but she still had stomach troubles. Then one day, Elena received intuitive guidance to drink peppermint tea. She began drinking it every day for a week, and, to her amazement, it stopped all her nausea and pain!

Elena now recommends peppermint to anyone with stomach complaints. She is careful to use only good-quality herbs from the health-food store. Sometimes she adds the fresh leaves in her hot teas or in refreshing iced teas in the warmer months. Elena is pleased that Divine guidance healed her stomach.

Recommended Herbs

Consider whether any of the following herbs may be of use to you on your own healing journey. If you have a pre-existing condition or are currently on any medications or treatment plans, please get advice from your care provider before adding herbs to your regimen.

While I (Robert) love the effect of herbal formulas, the taste is usually not the most pleasant. Before taking liquid extracts and tinctures, I always dilute them in water and have a "chaser" ready. I usually use a half cup of water, but I know some people use a mere tablespoon and drink it in one mouthful. It doesn't matter how much water you mix with the herbal medicines—just make sure you drink it all. Then quickly follow with another drink, perhaps juice.

It is best to take herbal medicines just after eating, unless the directions state otherwise. You don't need to be exact, but don't wait longer than 30 minutes or it may give you digestive upset.

Ginger (*Zingiber officinale*)

Ginger is a common spice with a warming flavor that you've likely used in cooking. You can use ginger for healing as well. Consider preparing your meals with the idea of healing pain. Include fresh ginger in stir-frys, soups, and even juices.

This root's warmth helps clear old, low energy by pushing out the blocks in your body that hold on to pain. In herbal medicine, ginger is one of the most effective anti-inflammatory plants. It relaxes muscular tension and takes away joint pain. It also stimulates your circulation and assists the transport of helpful cells around your body.

A study published in the journal *Arthritis* compared the effectiveness of ginger to that of cortisone and ibuprofen when used in the treatment of osteoarthritis and rheumatoid arthritis. This particular study found that an extract of ginger was as effective an anti-inflammatory agent as cortisone, and the ibuprofen had no effect on cytokine production, one of the factors that causes pain. Cortisone has a long list of possible side effects, including weight gain, depression, severe headaches, chest pains, and sleeping issues. Ginger, on the other hand, has very few side effects, although it should be avoided before surgery and by those with peptic ulcers, due to its blood-thinning quality.

Research conducted at Odense University in Denmark also found ginger to be a highly effective healer. The study gave arthritic patients a small amount of ginger each day for three months. Almost all the participants experienced significant improvements in pain levels, swelling, and morning stiffness just by eating ginger. The head researcher, Dr. Srivastava, went on to say that ginger is superior to nonsteroidal anti-inflammatory drugs (NSAIDs). These drugs only work to block the production of inflammatory markers. Ginger does this and also reduces existing inflammation.

Taking ginger as a liquid tincture can alleviate nausea and other digestive discomforts. Take 10 drops in a little water, and within 15 minutes, the complaint will dissipate. For chronic pain and inflammation, you may need higher amounts. In these cases, take 25 drops of ginger tincture three times per day.

Ginger in liquid form contains alcohol, so avoid taking too much. A safer method for higher doses is tablets or capsules. Your body can handle a higher concentration; try 1,000 mg, divided into two or three doses, per day. After a couple of weeks, you'll find pain and inflammation decreasing.

Boswellia (*Boswellia serrata*)

Boswellia is a resin that's produced from a type of frankincense tree. True frankincense resin has a long history of being used for its cleansing and uplifting properties, often as an incense. It's smoldered over charcoal to rid the space of negative energies and welcome in the angels. Boswellia emits a similar vibration.

A 2003 randomized, double-blind study compared the efficacy of boswellia with a placebo in patients with osteoarthritis. After a period of eight weeks, the groups were tested for pain, then the control and the treatment groups were switched. At the end of the trial, it was clear that when patients used boswellia, they noticed a decrease in pain and swelling, an increase in flexibility, and general improvement in comfort levels. The researchers suggest that boswellia could be a viable treatment for arthritis patients.

In 2013 a medical research team tested a combination of boswellia and turmeric against celecoxib (brand name Celebrex) in patients with osteoarthritis. They found that the herbal combination was more effective at treating pain and inflammation than the celecoxib. They noted that the boswellia and turmeric combination was well tolerated and had no adverse effects.

Since boswellia comes from a resin, it's best taken as a tablet or capsule. Some manufacturers produce liquid formulas, but the oily taste makes it difficult to stick with. Take 4,000 mg, divided into two or three doses, per day.

Capsaicin

Capsaicin is the active component of chili peppers. Studies have shown that using a topical cream containing capsaicin can dramatically reduce the severity of pain. Arthritis sufferers have reported a marked improvement that can last for several weeks. The reason behind this is that capsaicin temporarily numbs the pain-sensitive nerve fibers. While these nerve endings repair, you remain pain-free!

You can find creams containing capsaicin at health-food stores. Apply it two to four times per day, and after about two weeks you should notice an improvement with painful arthritis or sore muscles. This cream works by stimulating, then decreasing, pain signals in your body.

To make your own potent, capsaicin-infused oil, add 2 tablespoons of dried organic chili flakes to 1 cup of organic, cold-pressed, extra-virgin olive oil. Place the mixture in a double boiler on the stove, or in a heatproof bowl sitting over a pot of boiling water. Heat gently for 60 minutes, allowing the chili to infuse the oil. Strain by pouring through some muslin into a clean jar, allow to cool, then cover tightly.

Please take every precaution to keep this oil away from your eyes and mouth, and out of the reach of children. To use, apply a small amount (a couple of drops) to the affected area, and gently rub in. You may want to wear gloves when applying, to avoid irritation. It's normal to experience heat and light redness, but if you sense that it's too irritating, then remove it as soon as possible.

Arnica

The herb arnica is harmful if consumed in its raw form. Homeopathic arnica, however, is highly effective at treating bruising, pain, and swelling. The exact mechanisms by which it works are unknown, but research has shown it to be especially good for acute injuries and postsurgery swelling.

To make a homeopathic remedy, there are a series of dilutions (known as *potentizations).* Let's use arnica as our example: 1 drop of arnica extract added to 9 drops of solution (alcohol, water, or glycerol), then potentized (shaken), makes Arnica 1X. One drop of Arnica 1X added to 9 drops of solution, then potentized, makes Arnica 2X. This process continues until the desired level is reached. There is also a C scale—1 drop of arnica extract added to 99 drops of solution makes Arnica 1C, 1 drop of Arnica 1C added to 99 drops of solution makes Arnica 2C, and so on.

After you reach 12C, there is no longer any physical arnica remaining in the product, but the potentizations extract its energy to create a high-vibrational remedy. The magic of homeopathy removes the harmful aspects of an object while enhancing the healing properties. The process of serial dilution can continue many more times, to reach hundreds or thousands of dilutions. Paradoxically, the more "diluted" the remedy is, the more potent its energy becomes. Those higher dilutions affect the mental and emotional aspects of a person, whereas the lower potencies treat the physical.

Arnica is best taken when there's a recent injury or bruising, such as when you've fallen, tripped, or collided with something—for example, jamming a finger in a car door or hitting it with a hammer.

Homeopathy is not advised as a preventive measure. We have heard of a football team who took arnica before a match with the idea that it would decrease recovery time, heal injuries, and get them back on the field faster. Instead, the opposite happened, and they bruised terribly!

Remember, homeopathy is based on the principle of "like cures like." So a substance that causes symptoms in a healthy individual will heal those same symptoms for someone who's unwell. And a homeopathic remedy can create the symptoms in healthy individuals that it cures in the sick or injured. Indeed, some people are actually employed to take homeopathic remedies just to see what the remedy can treat.

While the reasons behind arnica's efficacy are unknown, the results cannot be ignored. Consider homeopathic arnica a first-aid remedy in your cupboard.

Willow Bark (*Salix alba*)

Willow bark is a time-tested, traditional remedy. It can reduce fever, lower inflammation, and alleviate pain anywhere in the body. It is available for purchase as a tea, a liquid extract, or tablets.

A study conducted on 200 patients with back pain found that those given willow bark showed marked improvement over the placebo group, and the group given a higher dosage of willow bark found even more relief than the low-dosage group. It is an excellent herb for osteoarthritis because it reduces both the sensation of pain and the inflammation that aggravates it.

One reason why willow bark is effective at reducing inflammation is that it contains salicin. This compound was extracted during the 1800s to develop acetylsalicylic acid, more commonly known as aspirin. Willow bark does not work as quickly as aspirin, but its effects may last longer. And while aspirin does bring about very quick, effective pain relief and fever reduction, overuse can lead to digestive issues and stomach complaints. Interestingly, the original version, willow bark, can also heal digestive inflammation and is much better tolerated.

It is interesting to note that one double-blind, placebo-controlled trial suggested that the pain-relieving properties of willow bark could not be attributed to the salicin alone. So when you take a medicine that isolates that substance, you lose out on the other healing powers of the herb. Truly, the whole is always greater than the sum of its parts!

Turmeric (*Curcuma longa*)

Turmeric has been dubbed one of the most effective plant-based medicines for inflammation of all kinds. It is able to ease swelling throughout the entire body and also target specific areas of pain. If you treat the symptoms of pain without addressing the inflammation, the swelling and pressure builds so that the pain will return as soon as you stop taking the medicine. When you clear the inflammation, you are also targeting the cause of your pain.

Turmeric is a culinary spice that's often used to add color to dishes. However, the magical properties of this orange root go far beyond its ability to brighten the look of a dish. Turmeric contains a compound called curcumin. This natural chemical has been researched dozens of times and continues to show more amazing pain-reducing qualities. Turmeric can be used for osteoarthritis, rheumatoid arthritis, backaches, menstrual discomfort, headaches, and any other inflammatory condition. It is also wonderful for liver detoxification.

An Indian study conducted in 2013 showed the efficacy and safety of using turmeric for pain management and healing.

One hundred twenty patients with osteoarthritis were given either a placebo, turmeric extract, glucosamine, or a combination of glucosamine and turmeric. The group that showed the most improvement on a number of clinical assessments was the one given turmeric.

Turmeric has a more potent reaction in the body when it's consumed alongside some kind of fat. A traditional preparation would be a curry dish that contains the spice as well as coconut cream. You might also try mixing turmeric into a smoothie with coconut oil, or adding a teaspoon to yogurt. Select organic soy, almond, or dairy yogurt, and be sure not to use a low-fat or fat-free version!

Some companies are creating turmeric preparations to ensure that they contain a standardized level of curcumin. This can be good because it allows you to know that you're getting the amount that research suggests is the most effective. On the other hand, you're taking a product that's now unbalanced and unlike the way God created it. We prefer to trust in God's wisdom and know that everything was created perfect, so we don't feel the need to take standardized supplements. Instead, seek whole products that are as nature intended.

Turmeric is an excellent antioxidant, so it's often taken as a cancer preventive. Inflammatory conditions cause greater stress to the body, using up precious resources that the body may not be able to replenish as quickly as it needs to. This high demand can lead to cell mutations and damage and, eventually, cancer. Turmeric helps clear away inflammation and protect cells from oxidative damage.

Devil's Claw (*Harpagophytum procumbens*)

While the name isn't angelic, devil's claw is a highly effective remedy for pain. (The name is derived from the plant's appearance: spiky barbs in a circle look a lot like a scary claw!) Take devil's claw for 8 to 12 weeks to begin seeing improvements in joint flexibility and pain levels.

One study, conducted over four months on 122 people, compared devil's claw with a leading pain medication for arthritis. Those who took the herb reported as much pain relief as those taking the pharmaceutical drugs, but with fewer side effects. Another study compared 38 people who took devil's claw with 35 who took the pharmaceutical Vioxx for a year. Both groups experienced the same level of pain relief. However, it is important to note that Vioxx was removed from the market in 2004 because it was linked to an increased risk of heart attack and stroke. Devil's claw, on the other hand, has been used for hundreds of years and appears to be very safe and well tolerated.

I (Robert) prefer to give devil's claw as a liquid extract because I feel the liquid contains a higher energy than tablet and capsule preparations. Follow your own intuitive feelings, and see if you sense the same thing. I often prescribe ½ teaspoon (2.5 ml) three times per day. Remember, herbs in liquid form are best taken in a little water, just after eating.

Saint-John's-wort (*Hypericum perforatum*)

Saint-John's-wort is commonly thought of as a remedy for stress and depression. It is a wonderfully uplifting herb that raises your body's serotonin levels naturally. By increasing these feel-good hormones, you experience more joy in your day. This alone could be wonderfully healing, because the fastest way to a pain-free body is to find happiness first!

Along with raising your energy and vitality, Saint-John's-wort also treats nerve pain. This type of pain may be sharp, stabbing, and sudden; feel like pins and needles; or even resemble a sense of numbness. And, according to a 2013 study published in the journal *Phytomedicine*, Saint-John's-wort helps block pain pathways and is a great treatment for migraines.

This herb can also be of service to people who have endured amputations and experience the "phantom pain" caused by nerve signals being misinterpreted. I (Robert) recall one patient who had a finger removed, yet she could still feel tingling in that fingertip, with desperate urges to scratch it. After a few weeks of taking Saint-John's-wort, she happily reported that the annoyance was gone.

We adore working with the herbal extract of Saint-John's-wort, particularly as a liquid or tincture. A good-quality product will be a rich, deep red color; this is symbolic of the protection and security it gives. There's something so valuable in Saint-John's-wort extract. It's akin to happiness in a bottle. It pulls you away from chaos and drama, and lifts you up so you gain a new perspective on how to heal. However, these qualities are only present in the liquid form; it appears the tablets and capsules are missing this energetic component. Take 7 drops, three times per day. Within the week, your soul will feel refreshed. You will start smiling more, and pain will ease. Continue taking Saint-John's-wort for two or three months, or as you feel guided.

The homeopathic formulation is wonderful, too; try Hypericum 12C for nerve pain.

As soon as you take Saint-John's-wort, Archangel Raphael works with you and guides you on your healing journey. He will show you ways of changing your posture and sleeping habits to make your body more comfortable. Trust your intuitive feelings and be courageous in making the necessary changes.

Another of my (Robert's) patients had chronic backaches. He was in constant pain and was often hunched over in severe discomfort. He worked as a water delivery person, carrying large, heavy bottles into offices and homes every day. After he took Saint-John's-wort, his discomfort eased, his posture improved, and he recognized that his job was causing him more harm than good. The pay wasn't worth the physical agony. His angels guided him to a job opportunity as an ambulance officer, so now *he* guides others to a long and healthy life.

Cautionary Note: Saint-John's-wort has significant interactions with certain medications, including some antidepressants, statins, and oral contraceptives. If you are currently taking medication, consult with your health-care practitioner before taking Saint-John's-wort.

Cramp Bark (*Viburnum opulus*)

While cramp bark has not yet been subject to scientific study, it has a long history of success and has proven its healing power in the hands of many herbalists. As the name suggests, cramp bark allows your muscles to release their tension.

As you take cramp bark, you are able to let go. Tension, old emotions, pain, discomfort, and judgments simply fall away. It's a wonderful herb, and it begins work immediately. Take just 10 drops, three times per day, and you'll feel a difference.

Your body has an innate intelligence and knows the priorities of your healing journey. We call this "the direction of cure." Naturally, your body wants to heal your internal organs before worrying about skin conditions—even if that rash is the bane of your existence! In the same way, your body focuses on healing your mental and emotional concerns before delving into your physical ones. This makes absolute sense: if you're depressed, or even suicidal, would having a pain-free back make you happier? At first, you might say, "Absolutely!" But perhaps those heavy emotions triggered the back pain to begin with.

Cramp bark helps takes you through the direction of cure. It will connect you to your Higher Self and determine exactly what needs releasing first. If you start taking it and have a sudden desire to speak with an old friend, trust that notion. It may trigger a profound healing.

Everyone walks a unique path, so we cannot say to you the exact way cramp bark will affect you. This is why science has struggled with this herb—it works on another level that's more than simple chemicals and compounds. It has a higher intelligence that speaks to your body on a deep level.

Corydalis (*Corydalis ambigua*)

Corydalis is said to be one of the strongest pain relievers in all of herbal medicine. Studies have shown it to be effective against inflammatory, acute, and chronic pain. It is a member of the poppy family, like opium—but without the harmful side effects or danger of addiction. One researcher found corydalis to have 10 percent of the potency of opium (which is significant!), with pain relief lasting up to two hours.

This is a hard tuberous root that takes much effort to break down into a powder, signaling it's best used for hard pain cases, when other herbs have failed. It's effective at relieving many types of pain, including arthritis, back, neck, and menstrual pain. Studies suggest that the pain-relieving compound in corydalis does not lose effectiveness over long periods of use, unlike other opiates such as morphine, so it truly is a wonder for chronic pain. Of course, always check to ensure it won't interfere with other medications.

We suggest using this herb for a month or two to control your symptoms. Then move on to something else that can support you in a different way. Corydalis stops pain, but you mustn't rely on it. We don't recommend taking corydalis for more than three months. Energetically, herbs want to be with you only for the short-term. After clearing pain from your body, they're no longer needed. They are not meant to be preventive treatments.

Start with a large dose of 2 teaspoons (10 ml). Then, for the first week, take ½ teaspoon (2.5 ml), three times a day, and slowly decrease your dose each day thereafter. Your ego may try to convince you that this will bring back the pain, but remember that herbal medicines are different from pharmaceutical pain relievers. Herbs work with your system in a holistic way to repair and strengthen rather than simply masking the symptoms. The pain will be removed from your aura, so when you stop taking the herbs, you will continue to feel wonderfully comfortable in your precious body.

Recommended Supplements

We have found the following supplements to be very helpful for many people in the management of their pain. As we've said, if you have a pre-existing condition or are currently on any medications or treatment plans, please get advice from your care provider before taking any supplements.

Take supplements with food, unless otherwise stated in the directions. It is usually best to ingest supplements just before eating (unlike herbal remedies, which are best taken *after* eating).

SAMe (S-Adenosyl Methionine)

SAMe is one of my (Robert's) favorite treatments for depression, grief, and stress. It works incredibly fast, and I often compare it to a light switch—it illuminates the room by casting out all darkness. I've seen this product help people in their darkest moments and lift the spirits of depressed patients in a matter of days. When you take SAMe, the world becomes a brighter place. You laugh more, and it's a real, genuine laughter.

SAMe is also wonderful for clearing pain, although its mechanisms for doing so are not clearly understood. Some SAMe is naturally produced in the body. Taking it as a supplement seems to reduce inflammation and boost feel-good hormones. Studies have shown SAMe to be as effective as some NSAIDs (nonsteroidal anti-inflammatory drugs), without the common side effects or cardiovascular risks that other drugs can have. One of the only possible issues with SAMe is its rather high price. SAMe is a very unstable product, requiring that many quality-control procedures be put in place, which drives up the cost. Trust us, though—it is well worth it!

Dosage is key when it comes to SAMe. Due to the high manufacturing costs, many retail products have only low levels of the compound. Keep in mind that you will need 800 to 1,200 mcg per day to feel relief. (This is done in divided doses, 400 mcg two or three times per day.) Most SAMe pills are enterically coated to prevent them from being broken down in the stomach; instead, they are broken down in the small intestine. Therefore, it is important not to break tablets apart, as this will cause degradation.

Good-quality SAMe products will contain cofactors to help the absorption, such as zinc and B vitamins. Although you will want high amounts of SAMe, you may not want too much of the other ingredients in the supplement. Check with a health-care professional or naturopath for recommendations.

Cautionary Note: SAMe is known to interact with some drugs, including antidepressants, and is not recommended for certain conditions, such as bipolar disorder. Consult a qualified care professional before taking this supplement.

Omega-3s

Omega-3 fatty acids can be found in fish oil and certain plant oils. Omega-3s are considered "essential" fats because your body cannot make them; you must consume them in your diet. Fish oil contains the omega-3s docosahexaenoic acid (DHA) and eicosapentaenoic acid (EPA). Some plant oils contain alpha-linolenic acid (ALA), which your body may convert to DHA and EPA.

There are countless studies supporting the use of fish oil for treating pain. It lubricates the joints and reduces inflammation in the body. Many people have found that after taking fish oil for a few months, they can reduce, or totally eliminate, their need for pain medications. Be sure to read labels to make sure you are getting enough omega-3s. You may need 2,000 mg of EPA per day, or more, depending on your health and physical condition. However, the source of fish oil can play a role in its health properties. For example, if it is derived from large fish like tuna, mackerel, or cod, then there can be unacceptably high levels of mercury present.

A healthy, mercury-free choice is flaxseed or linseed oil. (They're different names for the same thing.) As mentioned, these oils contain ALA, which your body breaks down and converts into EPA and DHA. Flaxseed oil supplements are usually made up of 52 to 62 percent omega-3s, whereas fish oil is only 30 percent. It is better for both your body and the environment to consume flaxseed oil. You can purchase it as liquid or capsules; just note that some brands must be stored in the fridge to avoid going rancid. The ideal dose is two teaspoons per day, or 10,000 mg divided into two or three doses.

MSM (Methylsulfonylmethane)

MSM is a sulfur compound that has been used to treat a wide range of conditions. It appears to block the message of pain along your nerve fibers. It can help with swelling, inflammation, and fluid by enhancing your body's natural anti-inflammatory compounds. Some feel that MSM can prevent the breakdown of cartilage, which is important in terms of lasting relief and long-term improvement for arthritis sufferers. One trial showed a 25 percent reduction in pain and a 30 percent improvement in range of movement in patients given MSM over three months.

Suggested doses to begin with are 1.5 to 3 g per day; then build up to 3 g twice daily for more intense pain.

Magnesium

Magnesium is used by the body in a number of diverse roles, including nerve function, blood glucose control, and blood pressure regulation. Magnesium is also used in every single muscle contraction, so the more you exercise, the more you need. (This is why it is highly recommended that athletes take it.) Although people often think of using this supplement only for muscle cramps, magnesium also eases general tension in your body and can help manage pain in a number of ways.

Many pain sufferers report terrible sleep patterns, and often toss and turn at night. Magnesium helps calm your nervous system and promotes restorative slumber. While it does not induce sleep, it does allow your body to relax enough to help you drift off and get the healing rest you need. As a general guideline, we recommend eight hours of sleep each night, so that you spend enough time in the deeper, restorative states, which can't be reached within a short period of time.

Magnesium also helps block NMDA receptors, which are important components in processing pain in your brain. So if you're deficient in this mineral, your pain response is more exaggerated. Consider increasing your intake of magnesium if you're highly sensitive and even the slightest bump can cause you agony.

We suggest 400 mg of elemental magnesium per day. We've found that it's best to take the supplement in the evening, because research shows that its absorption levels peak six hours after consumption. So if you take it before you sleep, you'll wake up with perfect levels and a greater tolerance for pain. Your body will be processing the messages of discomfort in a more balanced and healing way.

Vitamin D

We usually think of vitamin D for bone strength, yet science is showing us that it is important for our immune system, hormone levels, and even skin health. A study conducted in 2009 found that people with vitamin D deficiency required twice as much pain medication as those with regular levels. Therefore, if you've experienced chronic pain, please consider a vitamin D screening. This will quickly show whether supplementation is right for you.

The most natural form of vitamin D comes from sunlight. Spend a few minutes outdoors each day. (Be sure to choose times of day when you won't burn, and use a good natural sunscreen the rest of the time.) Allow the healing effects of the sun to shine into your soul. The rays have traveled a great distance to reach you. Your skin absorbs the sun's vitality, illuminating the healing potential of your body. Your body knows the best way to heal, and it will guide you through this journey. As you listen to your inner voice and the voice of your angels, you will be led down the path that's perfect for you.

If you choose to take supplements, be sure that they are of high-quality and plant-based origins. (Most vitamin D comes from lanolin, which is extracted from sheep's skin. The other main source is cod liver.) They work best when combined with a fat, so many supplements now include a little oil in the capsules to assist absorption. If yours does not, then take it with a teaspoon of coconut oil for the best effect.

Start by taking 1,000 IU per day, then have your levels checked in three months. If your vitamin D levels are not balanced at this point, speak with your health-care professional about another approach.

∾

Herbs and supplements are wonderful for healing pain, but you must also look at your body as a whole. You can't build a foundation for true wellness without addressing nutrition, which we will discuss in the next chapter.

∾ ∽

CHAPTER FIVE

Nutrition
to Conquer
Inflammation
and Pain

What you eat and drink is just as important to your health as what medicines you take and what therapies you undergo. As we said, if you address your pain on only a superficial level, you will not experience complete wellness. When you work on yourself in a holistic way, the angels support you and provide you with magical experiences.

The most optimal diet for your body consists of natural foods, mainly organic fruits and vegetables. You might think, *That sounds like what my great-grandmother ate!* Well, you'd be right. Looking back 100 years, organic food wasn't special—because that was all that existed!

Mother Nature created food perfectly. We don't need to alter the genetic makeup of plants or adulterate them with man-made chemicals. But now we grow things under such conditions that poisonous pesticides and harsh chemical fertilizers are often used. The food is laced with toxic coatings so it lasts longer on the shelf and more can be produced. Yet few consider the harmful effects all this has on the human body.

Your logical brain might try to convince you that eating organic produce is too expensive. However, when you avoid the processed garbage and choose real, natural food, you will remember how good you can feel when enjoying natural foods. You and your family will not only enjoy the tastes but also the feelings you receive. Instead of leaving fruit to wither in a bowl, your family will eat it and desire more. They can tell on a subconscious level that this food is healing from the inside out.

Maintaining the Acid-Alkaline Balance in Your Body

A low-acidic diet is a wonderful way to release chronic inflammation from your body. Acid-causing foods produce just that—metabolic acids. Too much of these can lead to general discomfort along with other health concerns. Many people have found dramatic improvements just by altering what they eat to support an alkaline state.

Rheumatoid arthritis is one of the most responsive conditions to a low-acid diet. Furthermore, many of my (Robert's) patients have found relief from their symptoms by ceasing to eat foods from the nightshade family, which contain inflammation-inducing alkaloids. Members of this group include potatoes, tomatoes, chilis, and eggplant.

Even normal metabolic processes can create acids that need to be cleared. For example, exercise can create a buildup of lactic acid; most people have experienced the soreness that results a day or two after a workout. Similar pain is happening on a smaller scale with acid that floats through your system. If enough builds up, then you will feel it more consciously.

Arthritis and general stiffness in your joints is caused by acids that lodge themselves in those areas. Osteoarthritis is characterized by a decline in cartilage in the joints; this can occur anywhere, including the fingers, knees, hips, neck, and back. This is partly caused by general wear and tear, but trapped acids will also exacerbate the sensation of pain. Eating a diet that shifts your body into an alkaline state will help flush them out.

Not only do acidic foods create inflammation, but they can actually pull calcium out of your skeleton. This makes your bones brittle and more prone to breaks. The enamel on your teeth can also become more fragile, which is something that cannot be repaired. If you show signs of low bone density, such as osteoporosis or osteopenia, then please check your diet.

It would be wise to research a full list of alkaline and acidic foods. To start with, simply keep in mind that most leafy greens and fruits are alkaline, as are root and cruciferous vegetables. Good foods to incorporate into your diet include garlic, apple cider vinegar, cayenne pepper, cinnamon, ginger, and almonds. Acid-producing substances to avoid include fried foods, animal meats, sugar, dairy, refined cereals, white flour, artificial sweeteners, coffee, soda, and alcohol.

Lemons for Alkalinity

While it might seem natural to think that citrus fruits would be acid-causing in your body, they actually convert in your system to promote an alkaline state. Lemon is one of those magical foods that can assist in many different health areas. It is highly antioxidant, protects cells from damage, prevents abnormal cell growth, and can reduce inflammation. Enjoy half a fresh, organic lemon squeezed into a glass of warm water first thing in the morning to kick-start your digestion and help your body rid itself of acids.

If you have a high-powered blender or juicer, you can use the entire lemon, peel and all, rather than only the juice. Just make sure you've rinsed the lemon really well first. However, the flavor can take some adjusting to, so you may want to start off with just a slice or two in your water. Once you are able to tolerate the taste, you can add more, until you can include a whole lemon daily. It is incredibly cleansing; you will feel lighter and clearer after just a few days.

Increasing Endorphins, Your Body's Pain Medicine

When you are hurt, your body releases its own pain reliever: endorphins. This neurotransmitter blocks the pathway of pain at the brain stem and is a naturally occurring substance that has an opiate-like effect, rather like morphine. The more endorphins floating around your body, the less pain you will experience.

Endorphins are produced from amino acids, which are natural compounds that you need for wellness. Your body can synthesize some of these, but others must be gained from your diet. When you consume high-protein foods, your body breaks them down into the complete range of amino acids.

Good vegan sources of protein include:

- Soy (organic, to avoid chemicals and genetically modified soy)
- Rice protein (organic only)
- Pea protein
- Almonds (including almond milk and butter)
- Quinoa
- Lentils
- Beans

Good non-vegan sources of protein, to be consumed in moderation, include:

- Dairy
- Eggs (from free-range chickens)
- Whey protein

Choose only organic, non–genetically modified options, and make sure you're eating protein at every meal to give you adequate amino acids. Also, consuming a wide range of organic fruits and vegetables will help nourish your system in a gentle way.

If your diet doesn't provide you with enough amino acids, you may need to take supplements for a short period of time. Phenylalanine is an essential amino acid, and excellent for pain-management support because it helps prevent the breakdown of endorphins, thereby prolonging their effect. There are two kinds: *D* and *L*. L-phenylalanine is the natural version found in proteins, while D-phenylalanine is synthesized in a lab. L-phenylalanine is more readily absorbed; however, it can be overstimulating in sensitive people, so pay close attention to your moods, anxiety levels, and heart rate. Start with 500 mg twice daily. Then, if your body can tolerate it, consider moving up to three times per day for one month only, before reducing to 500 mg once a day. You should notice dramatic changes in your pain levels within the first week.

Please understand that phenylalanine supplementation is not a true cure. Instead, it adjusts your reactions to the sensation of pain. The underlying dysfunction may still be present, but you will be better able to direct your true healing once your symptoms are under control. So look at this as a short-term management strategy while simultaneously working on the cause of pain.

Allergies and Dietary Intolerances

If you eat large amounts of any food, your body will get tired of them. Indeed, you can develop an intolerance to anything! If you eat tomatoes for every meal, you may very well end up having bad reactions to them one day. This is why naturopaths have long advised their clients about implementing a rotational diet. After eating something, you would be wise to avoid it for several days. Ensure that you try new foods all the time. Don't get stuck on one type of meal and the same ingredients. We all have our favorites, but we also need to be mindful of what is optimal for our bodies.

Consuming something to which you are allergic leads to inflammation. This can cause all sorts of health issues—soreness, fatigue, headaches, and skin complaints—but it also leads to the production of endorphins. It is a tricky situation your body puts you in. On the one hand, the allergen is doing damage to your system. On the other hand, it causes you to produce endorphins, which make you feel good—so your body wants more! It is easy to develop an unhealthy relationship to a substance to which you are allergic. Recognize that these feel-good hormones are only being produced in order to help your body cope with the damage that your diet is causing.

Releasing Unhealthy Food Habits with the Help of Your Angels

Call upon your angels to help you rid yourself of any unhealthy addictions. In our previous book *Angel Detox,* we noted that everyone who prays for help when giving up a food or beverage receives Divine intervention. Help may not come as an obvious sign at first, yet eventually the cravings are released. People are able to let go of foods and drinks that they have failed to give up in the past. After calling on the support of their angels, they are able to kick these items out of their lives for good!

To enlist the angels to help you, find a quiet space where you won't be disturbed. Begin by focusing on your breathing, and relax your mind. As you feel more comfortable, say either aloud or in your mind:

"Dear God, Jesus, and Archangel Raphael, I call upon your assistance now. Please be here with me as I make this commitment to my health. I wish to banish all pain from my life; to do so, I know I need to release these addictions. Please guide me through this healing process. I trust you and know that you have only my highest good in mind. Thank you."

Now visualize the items you wish to release hovering above your stomach. You may clairvoyantly see thin, spiderweb-like cords linking those foods and beverages to your body. Raphael's emerald-green healing energy will dissolve the cords, cutting these addictions out of your life.

You may notice sensations running through your body; perhaps you will *feel* Raphael clearing your pain. Regardless of whether you're consciously experiencing any particular sensations, the healing is taking place. The angels simply need your permission to intervene into your life. Once they have this, they can work their healing miracles. From this point on you will have Archangel Raphael by your side, guiding you on how to live a pain-free life.

Archangel Raphael is our supreme healer who never judges us for our habits. He will work with you compassionately to release any unhealthy items. You'll simply let go of them, never considering them as options again. It's possible that you might have one last binge, then never look back. Or you may find that your tastes change, and you no longer experience the same cravings. However it occurs, trust that Divine intervention is at work and your angels are with you.

You may also notice differences when going out to eat with friends and family. While you may have ordered other menu items in the past, now you will want more natural, nutritious choices. You will find new inspiration in your cooking at home and create wonderful-tasting dishes. Your inner voice will be awakened, and you'll know the angels are in play.

The Healing Power of Water

The average person can survive for weeks without food, but only a few days without water. It is vital to keeping you healthy, happy, and pain-free. Through general metabolic processes, your body loses over a liter (4.2 cups) of water each day. When you don't drink enough to replenish this loss, your body holds on to as much as fluid as possible, making it a challenge to reduce swelling. The more you drink, the easier it is for your system to flush out toxins and inflammatory compounds.

Your brain is the center of your nervous system, and it needs water to work properly. Staying hydrated is essential to keeping your bodily functions running smoothly. Otherwise, you will find yourself fatigued and unable to concentrate. It will become harder to focus on positive and loving thoughts, your mood may become depressed, and your connection to the angels may be strained. By providing your body and brain with the water you need, you'll enjoy light thoughts and a stable bond with the angelic realm.

People often misinterpret thirst as hunger and eat instead of providing their bodies with essential water. When you think you feel "hunger," take a moment to tune in to your body. Have a glass of water, and see if the sensation goes away after five minutes. You may be surprised by how often water satisfies your cravings!

Measuring your water intake will allow you to ensure that you are regularly hydrating your system. Aim for a half ounce of water per pound of body weight, or 30 ml per kilogram. Get a stainless-steel or glass water bottle that you can take with you during your daily activities, and remember to regularly fill it.

You can make drinking water more fun by adding small amounts of freshly squeezed organic juice, or slices of fresh organic lemon and lime. Combine this with fresh organic mint leaves for a refreshing treat on a warm day.

The Quality of Your Drinking Water

While it is essential to consume adequate amounts of water, the quality of the source is also important for your health. Here's a simple experiment: Notice how often you need to visit the bathroom. After drinking a tall glass, do you feel the urge to relieve yourself only 30 minutes later? With better-quality water, you may not need to go for an hour or more, and when you do, you'll release less than what you drank. This is proof that the water didn't simply pass through your body and has instead been put to good use in vital metabolic processes.

Do your research into the quality of your region's tap water—you may be surprised by how poor it is. If you choose to drink bottled water, find out the process used to collect it; many brands are actually treated with chemicals. The best option is a natural springwater that involves minimal handling, taken from an underground source and put straight in the bottle. This will not have the harsh chemicals or pollutants that treated waters do. Unprocessed water retains the minerals and trace elements that your body needs. There are many reputable companies who provide at-home springwater dispensers. Be sure that the containers that hold the water are made of BPA-free plastic (we'll discuss the dangers of BPA in the next chapter).

Check the mineral analysis of your water to ensure that it doesn't have only sodium and chloride. While some sodium is needed, it shouldn't be the sole mineral present. Good-quality water will also include small traces of calcium, magnesium, and potassium, which help your body absorb and use the water you consume. This is why purified and distilled waters, while better than tap water, are still not ideal. They may sound "clean," but they have been processed to remove all of those minerals. There is a compromise: filter your water, but add the minerals back in with salt! Note, however, that most table salts have been refined, thereby stripping them of these minerals. It is important to use only good-quality Celtic, Atlantic, Himalayan, or Dead Sea salts. Just add a tiny pinch to your water bottle and shake well.

Maintaining Your Electrolyte Balance Naturally

Electrolytes are special minerals that your body needs for nerve and muscle function, hydration, regulating blood pH and blood pressure, and rebuilding damaged tissue. You lose electrolytes through your sweat, and when you are deficient, you can experience pain, muscle twitching, and light-headedness.

I (Robert) would experience these symptoms after hard workouts at the gym. At first I thought I was deficient in magnesium, so I used a high-quality supplement for several weeks. There was a slight change, but I still had aches and pains that wouldn't go away. I felt like I was doing more harm at the gym than good. Intuitively I knew there was something else going on.

My naturopathic dispensary is well stocked, so I have a vast array of supplements and herbal medicines at my disposal. However, my angels were telling me that none of these were the answer to my situation. I meditated and prayed to Heaven for help figuring this one out. What was causing me so much discomfort and restless nights of tossing and turning?

The angels said I was running out of electrolytes. I trusted their message; after all, it makes sense! When you exercise, you sweat and thereby lose these valuable minerals. That's why sports drinks are fortified with them. However, I wasn't about to drink any artificially colored, flavored, sweetened "health drinks"! I started researching natural replacements, but there aren't really any commercially available supplements. There are several fruits rich in electrolytes, such as lemons and limes, so I began adding these to my morning juices and noticed a big difference in the way I felt.

The angels also guided me to use Himalayan salt. Himalayan, Celtic, Atlantic, and Dead Sea salts contain the electrolytes you need, and you need add only the smallest pinch to your water bottle. It shouldn't taste super salty, and you could always add more flavor with a slice of lemon or lime, which also packs in even more benefits.

I find that when I work out now, I have greater endurance. My body is doing what my brain is telling it to, and I can have intense workout sessions without aching for the next few days. So please try maintaining your electrolyte balance naturally, and experience greater comfort within your body.

◌

It may sometimes seem challenging to make lifestyle changes, but it is for your own well-being. What are you willing to do to rid yourself of pain forever?

We follow many of the practices in this book ourselves and have heard touching testimonials from clients all around the world. When you make the effort, your life can change in miraculous ways. As you choose to heal, you allow the miracle to occur. By taking action steps and purifying your life of chemicals, you show the universe that you're serious about your wellness and are ready to live pain-free.

෧ ௸

CHAPTER SIX

DETOXING TO RELEASE PAIN

Your body is your vehicle on Earth. You must treat it well in order to get the best from it. If you continually put in poor-quality fuel, how can you expect to have the vitality you crave? It's just like your car—service it well and it will serve you well. In the act of detoxification, or detox, you remove substances from your life that negatively impact your vitality. Herbs and supplements are often taken during this time to assist in the cleansing process.

Toxins attract inflammation, which leads to pain and sickness. The process to address this is simple: clear away toxins and you'll clear away pain. You don't need to go on a harsh or overly restrictive cleanse. Indeed, you may find that you enjoy detoxing because your body feels so good afterward.

Let go of the substances that are causing you harm. Isn't it worth it? Right now your ego might be saying that you shouldn't "have to" do this. But what if you could just try? Rather than having to pump your body full of medications just to get through the day, wouldn't it be nicer to let go of unhealthy substances, habits, and even relationships? We think so. We are passionate about living clean and healthy lives because we have felt the benefits firsthand. Right now you may think that you're giving something up—but in reality, you're gaining so much more.

If you've taken pain pills for a long time, your liver needs to be cleansed. (We recommend herbs for doing so in this chapter.) However, it is important to note that a liver cleanse may push any medications you are on out of your system very quickly, which could exacerbate the condition you are taking them for. It's essential that you get support and supervision. Work with a trusted health-care professional who has a thorough understanding of your condition and medications, and also wants to see you totally pain-free.

Specific Herbal Medicines for Releasing Toxins

The following herbs are known for their ability to cleanse. Their action is sometimes called "alterative" or "depurative" in herbal medicine, which means that they clean the blood. They aid in detoxification by facilitating the elimination of waste products, and they prevent metabolic toxins from accumulating in the body. Clearing these toxins will get rid of inflammation.

Barberry (*Berberis vulgaris*) helps heal the stomach and brings strength and tone to the digestive system. This makes it harder for toxins to be absorbed into the bloodstream. It also stimulates the liver and helps the body flush out unwanted chemicals.

Barberry isn't a very pleasant-tasting herb. However, it appears to have the best healing effects when you are able to taste its bitterness. So, for maximum therapeutic benefit, take it mixed with water rather than strong-tasting juices.

Blue flag (*Iris versicolor*) releases toxic buildup in the lymphatic system and reduces inflammation. It helps the lymph, fluid in your body that is responsible for immunity, to more freely circulate. The toxins are then processed through the liver and cleared from the bowel. This herb also helps balance hydration and works well for chronic skin complaints.

Burdock (*Arctium lappa*) clears toxins from the body by releasing them through the urinary tract. It's effective for relieving aches and pains stemming from gout. It may help with acidic conditions like arthritis, pain during exercise, and inflammation. It pulls out old toxins and acids that have been stored in the body. These waste products can create skin issues, and this herb helps your body cleanse itself.

Cleavers (*Galium aparine*) is an herb that goes deep into the body to clear toxins from the intracellular matrix. Many cleansing herbs will remove toxins from the extracellular matrix, the fluid that surrounds your cells. Cleavers, however, removes wastes from inside the cells and helps your body release them.

This herb is extremely cleansing. It can purify old sources of pain that have been with you for years. However, it should also be approached slowly and gently. If you've never detoxed before, try other methods before trying cleavers. If your body is holding on to old metabolic wastes, you may experience symptoms and side effects from your detox.

Echinacea (*Echinacea angustifolia* or *Echinacea purpurea*) is one of the most well-known herbs in the world. It stimulates the immune system and sends white blood cells on the hunt for anything harmful. It circulates through the lymphatic system and helps move the flow of toxins out of the body. Then it supports your body to repair any damage.

Gotu kola (*Centella asiatica*) gently helps circulation reach the top of the head. It breaks down scar tissue, thereby reducing inflammation and increasing flexibility. It also balances the nervous system and brings about clarity because it nourishes the brain. (There are stories of ancient emperors eating a leaf of gotu kola each day and reaching the age of 200.)

Nettle (*Urtica dioica* or *Urtica urens*) is a very detoxifying herb. Its extracts contain vitamins and minerals that promote the production of healthy new blood cells. Nettle leaves your system through the skin, so be sure that you exercise when taking this herb so that you can release it through your sweat.

People have historically used nettle to remove toxins by whipping their bare skin with its stinging leaves. The blisters and rashes that ensued were thought to be toxins and wastes trying to come out. In fact, the needles on the leaves contain histamine, which creates a rash on the skin. Histamine is responsible for allergic responses, so modern medicine relies heavily on antihistamines to treat allergies. Interestingly, when nettle is taken as a tincture or tea, it relieves allergies and hay fever. That's yet another example of the wonders of Mother Nature.

Red clover (*Trifolium pratense*) clears toxins from the body and also regulates female hormones. This herb is excellent both during and after menopause. Irregular hormones can lead to changes in mood, energy, and vitality, which can cause you to lose focus and engage in unhealthy habits. Red clover brings balance where it's needed and ensures that you maintain excellent care of your beautiful body.

Yellow dock (*Rumex crispus*) removes toxins via the bowels. Use it in low doses, as higher amounts can have a laxative effect. It treats chronic skin complaints as well as toxic bowels, because if your body is unable to release toxins through the bowels, it reabsorbs them into the bloodstream, which can lead to skin issues. It's also useful for arthritis that results in painful, irritated skin around the joints.

Herbal Medicines for the Liver

If nothing seems to heal your pain, consider doing a liver cleanse. This organ stores old toxins and energies that might be preventing you from healing. It does this as an act of service to ensure the toxins don't cause you greater harm. However, when too much toxicity accumulates, it becomes an obstacle to curing pain. So if you're trying everything possible to relieve your discomfort, to no avail, then it's time to think outside the box and focus on your liver.

When cleansing your liver, you're best served if you get professional support. The regular detox kits in health-food stores and pharmacies aren't specific enough. And remember, if you're on other medications, a liver cleanse will try to clear them out. This may not be the case for you, but it's always best to double-check—remember, do no harm!

The liver is the primary organ of detoxification. Toxins are processed and metabolized by the liver so they can be safely removed. There are two phases of liver detox. In the initial phase, enzymes bind to toxins to make them water soluble. (Often, many environmental toxins are fat soluble, which makes it harder for the body to remove them.) Then, in the second phase, the toxins are combined with organic compounds and passed into bile. Your body then releases them through the bowels.

The liver is one of the only human organs that can regenerate. It can regrow to its original size if it's damaged or partly removed in surgery. This is an amazing and loving gift from God. Care for your liver for a happy, healthy life.

The following herbs are wonderful for liver detoxification.

Andrographis (*Andrographis paniculata*) is immune enhancing. It fights infections, especially those of the liver. It protects your precious liver from damage.

Barberry (*Berberis vulgaris*) aids in detoxing the body by promoting the production and flow of bile, which helps the body excrete toxins.

Blue flag (*Iris versicolor*) is used for digestive liver insufficiency, symptoms of which can include constipation, nausea, and headaches. Blue flag stimulates the secretion of bile in order to improve digestion.

Bupleurum (*Bupleurum falcatum*) protects the liver, reduces inflammation, and balances the immune system. It's wonderful for balancing autoimmune conditions that involve the liver.

Dandelion root (*Taraxacum officinale*) stimulates digestion. It triggers the liver to get to work, and promotes proper bowel function. The grounded energy of dandelion makes it excellent for detox because it prevents you from losing focus or becoming disheartened. Sometimes your detox journey is a long one, so if you persist, you'll be rewarded with wonderful opportunities for health.

Milk thistle or **St. Mary's thistle** (*Silybum marianum*) is the ultimate liver herb and is beneficial for all aspects of this organ's function. It encourages the liver to heal and restore itself, and prevents damage to it from drugs and toxins. Studies have proven milk thistle's protective qualities, even against poisons as strong as the death-cap mushroom. Many people take this herb before drinking alcohol, saying that it makes it more difficult to get drunk. Note that while this herb does help preserve the liver, this shouldn't be an excuse to ingest harmful substances or drink alcohol to excess.

Rosemary (*Rosmarinus officinalis*) improves memory and concentration by sending blood to your brain. It also encourages phase two of liver detox. This is an effective herb to use when detoxing your emotions. It supports your nerves while treating the toxins.

Schizandra or **shisandra** (*Schisandra chinensis*) nourishes the nerves and balances energy. It helps the liver to perform both phases of liver detoxification. Use this herb when you're stressed and fatigued but need to detox.

Turmeric (*Curcuma longa*) enhances both phases of liver detoxification and helps the body clear toxins through bile. It's also an excellent antioxidant and anti-inflammatory. This is a very healing and nutritious herb.

The effects of turmeric can be enhanced if taken with a fat. This might mean mixing the powder with coconut milk, oil, or organic yogurt before ingesting. In tablet or capsule form, take it with some form of good fat, such as a handful of organic almonds, an avocado, or some yogurt.

Liver-Cleansing Dandelion Root Tea

A simple measure to detoxing is to enjoy dandelion tea (sometimes called dandelion coffee). It nourishes your digestive system and triggers the liver to excrete all that it no longer needs. It is made from the root, as the leaf does very little for your liver.

This healing herbal infusion stimulates digestion and encourages proper liver function. It is a grounding herb that brings awareness back into the body. By drinking a cup or two per day, you can understand what your body truly wants. For example, you may crave carbohydrates if you are deficient in B vitamin, or crave sugar if you lack magnesium. Your body isn't actually asking you for low-nutrient carbohydrates in the form of bread and pasta, but the vitamins in whole grains and legumes.

The tea has a very earthy flavor. You can adjust the taste by using organic honey, agave syrup, or raw coconut syrup. Avoid adding refined sugar, artificial sweeteners, or milk to your infusion. While this may be different from the tea you're used to, think of it as medicine. The cup sitting in front of you will bring you greater health and offer insights into your body's needs.

All you have to do is add one teaspoon of organic dried dandelion root to one cup of boiling water. (You may also use roasted organic dandelion root for a different flavor.) Allow it to steep for ten minutes before tasting, and add natural sweetener if needed.

I (Robert) don't find the taste all that appealing, but the benefits are worth it. Personally, I prefer to let the tea cool a little before I drink it. That way it becomes a warm drink rather than a hot tea. You could also add a squeeze of lemon, but I encourage you to try it without any additions first.

Parasite Cleanse

Often, the triggers for undiagnosed pain are parasites. These organisms live on or in a person's body, getting their food at the expense of the host and causing a multitude of health complaints. Common symptoms are digestive disturbances and abdominal cramping. If you've visited another country or a tropical location, or if you've eaten raw or undercooked fish, it's possible that you have contracted parasites.

Parasites can do a lot of harm that's often missed. They not only siphon away nutrients from the body but also excrete toxic materials into the bloodstream. This can affect the nervous system, energy levels, and mood. The symptoms of parasite infection can mimic many other health concerns, such as unresponsive arthritis. If an arthritis sufferer finds no relief with conventional treatments, the problem may actually be parasites. Particular parasites can encase themselves within the sensitive fluid of your joints, causing damage and creating inflammation that leads to pain. They can also lodge themselves in muscles and create a generalized pain.

Many people associate parasites with overseas travel, but they are rampant within the developed world, too. There are over 2 million cases of giardiasis and over 1.5 million new cases of toxoplasmosis diagnosed each year in the United States. The *Toxoplasma gondii* parasite, which causes toxoplasmosis, has been linked with more extroverted and reckless behavior. The Centers for Disease Control and Prevention has found a link between infection rates and schizophrenia, as the parasite appears to influence behavior. Changes in personality are also associated with this parasite, with people's personalities changing more the longer they remain infected.

There are two common practices when treating parasites. The first is to use high doses of herbs to remove all living organisms. This is usually done for about a week. The second method is to take smaller amounts of the herbal medicines for longer, so that you target the living parasites as well as any eggs. We feel that a combination of the two is the most effective approach, starting with a high dose, then reducing after a week and continuing treatment for a month.

It's best to get support from a trusted practitioner. Your naturopath or herbalist will be able to formulate a personalized mixture for you. There are also some wonderful tablet and capsule preparations that combine high levels of the following herbs. You may be able to find some in your local health-food store, but your practitioner might be able to supply something a little stronger.

Black walnut (*Juglans nigra*) is great for removing intestinal worms.

Clove (*Syzygium aromaticum*) is the perfect herb for parasite cleansing, as it covers so many bases. It targets two phases of the parasite life cycle by ridding the body of the living organisms and penetrating the egg coatings. It's highly effective at removing stubborn parasites, breaking through the walls that some organisms protect themselves within.

Goldenseal (*Hydrastis canadensis*) has the ability to remove parasites only at high concentrations. The major healing benefit of this herb is to repair the lining of your digestive system. It strengthens your stomach and bowels so toxic materials cannot reach your bloodstream. It should form part of your cleanse, but it can be left until the end, when the parasites have been removed.

Myrrh (*Commiphora molmol*) tastes terrible but is great for clearing parasites. It's best used in high doses for short periods of time.

Wormwood (*Artemisia absinthium*), as the name suggests, is used for treating worms and other intestinal parasites. As a sensitive person, you may find you can only tolerate small amounts of this herb. Respected herbalist Matthew Wood suggests that only one drop of the tincture be used once or twice a week.

Chinese wormwood (*Artemisia annua*) is usually better tolerated. It is specifically used for travelers' diarrhea, which is likely the result of parasite infection.

Removing Toxins from Your Life

All your efforts to detox will ultimately be futile if you unknowingly continue putting toxins into your body. Carefully consider whether the following substances have a place in your healthy lifestyle.

Fluoride

Fluoride is a mineral that is added to most toothpastes as well as the drinking water of many cities, with the promise that it helps prevent tooth decay. However, when comparing data from countries that have fluoridated water and those that don't, there's no difference in the occurrence of decay. Today, activists are demanding that their local water districts stop adding fluoride into the water supply, saying it is a toxic heavy-metal by-product of the phosphate fertilizer industry.

If you have tried everything and your pain persists, consider whether you need to reduce your exposure to fluoride. It is a toxin that is known to accumulate in the body and cause damage to your nervous system. It can create joint pain and interfere with thyroid function. It may even be a mutagen, which is something that causes genetic damage that may lead to cancer. Some studies suggest that fluoride negatively affects brain development, and others have linked low levels of intelligence with higher levels of fluoride.

Toothpaste tubes bear warning labels that suggest calling poison control if too much is swallowed. Each year, numerous children develop gastrointestinal issues due to the fluoride they've ingested via toothpaste. Interestingly, the amount of fluoride in a pea-size amount of toothpaste is similar to that contained in a cup of tap water in most areas. On the one hand, we're told to drink it; on the other, we're told to contact the poison hotline.

For your oral hygiene, we highly suggest that you switch to natural, chemical-free, fluoride-free toothpastes that don't contain carrageenan. (Carrageenan is a common food additive made from algae or seaweed that's used as a binder, thickener, and stabilizer, which can contribute to inflammation.) You can also make your own toothpaste from organic coconut oil, food-grade peppermint oil, and pure baking soda. These ingredients are readily available at health-food stores. Simply mix them to suit your own taste levels, and use as you would ordinary toothpaste.

Learn where your water is coming from and if it contains fluoride by contacting your local water authority. You can also purchase testing kits online. The best way to remove fluoride from water is through distillation or reverse osmosis; you can have a reverse-osmosis filtration system fitted in your home, which would be an investment in your health. After all, even if you don't drink tap water, if the water you are using to shower and bathe in contains fluoride, it may still be affecting your health and well-being.

The Dangers of BPA

BPA, short for bisphenol A, is a hormone-disrupting compound that has been linked to many health concerns, including hormonal imbalances, liver abnormalities, and poor brain development in infants. It may contribute to painful conditions such as diabetes, obesity, breast cancer, heart disease, and infertility.

BPA is often in plastics, including water bottles, food containers, and the lining of canned goods, because it helps make them stronger. Always look for BPA-free products whenever you purchase plastics or canned goods, such as the brand Amy's Kitchen, which guarantees that their products are free from this compound.

Plastic bottles containing BPA leach the chemical into their contents, especially when heated, such as in a hot car or a grocery store's warm storeroom. So it is best to enjoy your water in glass or stainless steel containers. We recommend buying drinking water in glass rather than plastic bottles. Many stores carry a selection of brands, such as Voss.

Even your toothbrush needs to be considered, as you're putting this into your mouth two or three times daily. The brand Preserve, available for sale online and in health-food stores, is BPA-free.

(Preserve also has a recycling program in which you may mail in your old toothbrushes and receive credit toward their products; they use the materials to manufacture new toothbrushes.)

Detox from Unhealthy Relationships

You may find the need to release toxic relationships in order to heal pain. I (Robert) had a patient who complained of severe back pain. She was in extreme discomfort when she had to sit in a car. I treated her three times, and while she saw a slight improvement, the majority of the pain wasn't shifting. I intuitively felt that part of the pain was connected to her husband, but when I questioned her about their relationship, she quickly shut down the topic. I let it go and trusted that her angels would show her the answer.

The following week she met up with some friends for an outing, and she was very excited about the trip. She would have to be in a car for over two hours, and while usually she would be in agony after 15 minutes, her pain was totally absent! She had a completely comfortable and relaxing journey and enjoyed a wonderful time with her friends.

However, when this woman got in the car to go home, her pain began to return. The closer she got to home, the worse the pain became. At her next appointment, she told me that she noticed her pain was worse the closer she got to her husband. She came to this conclusion with the help of angels showing her the way.

We discussed her treatment options and did some healing surrounding her relationship. She was holding on to old insecurities and resentment of her husband's frequent golf trips. By releasing those thoughts and feelings, she found that her pain levels diminished and her relationship strengthened.

Think about the people you often surround yourself with. Do you commonly find yourself feeling defensive, upset, or criticized when you are with a particular person? Gently remove this person's toxic energy from your life, and surround yourself with more joyful, uplifting people! You will almost certainly feel immediate relief in your body.

Prescribe a Vacation and Schedule in Fun

After you have removed harmful substances from your body and toxic relationships from your life, think about what you want to replace them with. Taking some time to relax—whether it's a couple of days or a couple of weeks—can make a world of difference. Indeed, many people find their pain disappears when on vacation. It's only when they return home and slip into old habits that their pain levels increase.

So maybe now *is* the perfect time for you to take a vacation. You might have fights with your ego voice about reasons not to go, but this could be the perfect solution for your health. Imagine what it would feel like to get away from it all for just the weekend. If this vision makes you feel relaxed, that is confirmation that now is the time. Don't delay your healing by worrying about how you're going to make it happen. If your angels think that a break is the best choice for you, then the funds and arrangements will fall into place.

It is also important that you make joy a regular part of your life, not just something that you do while on vacation. When did you last take some time to indulge a hobby? If you struggle to think of what interests you have, then it shows that you've lost touch with a part of yourself! So take a moment now to think of what would bring you peace and tranquillity. Perhaps you enjoy gardening, sewing, reading, walking, painting, dancing—anything! You're special and unique, and your needs are unlike anyone else's on Earth. We must always honor our individuality, with treatment as much as with life.

Now schedule time for these activities every week. They shouldn't be something you do only occasionally; instead, make them a part of your routine. Wouldn't you feel better if you honored yourself by doing the things you love more often? Of course you would.

Call upon your angels by saying:

"Angels, please give me the time, money, transportation, and anything else I need to spend time doing the things I love. I know it will help my health and allow my light to shine more brightly. Thank you."

ᄋ ᄋ

CHAPTER SEVEN

Incorporating Exercise into Your Life

Our bodies are designed to move. If you live a sedentary life, your muscles, joints, and bones begin to suffer. If you've been enduring chronic pain, then you'll likely have reduced the amount you exercise and how often you participate in other activities. It can feel like there's a big red stop sign in front of you. Pain halts your progress and limits your abilities . . . if you let it!

Engaging in gentle movements allows your body to find its perfect state of balance. Without it, you can become tense and stressed, and experience more discomfort than usual. The voice of pain will tell you that you must rest and avoid movement at all costs. In some situations this is good advice; however, the majority of the time, this puts your healing on hold.

Archangel Raphael can help you in your journey by giving you motivation to exercise. As we mentioned earlier, you can do far more for your health by improving your diet than by working out alone. However, as your vitality improves and you listen to your inner guidance, you'll naturally seek more movement. You'll want to exercise because it makes your body feel so good. Activity causes your body to release endorphins, those happy hormones that uplift your soul. Daily exercise can also help you clear through depression, fatigue, and feelings of loneliness.

Sometimes you may receive healing guidance when exercising. For example, one of our readers, Kevin Hunter, enjoyed working out and feeling the benefits in his body and mind. One day, as he was jogging home from the gym, he felt a strain near his ankle. He tried to walk it off; however, he limped and felt a sharp pain each time his foot landed on the pavement. He still had quite a distance before he reached home, and he wondered how he would make it.

Suddenly, Kevin heard a voice reminding him, "Ask for help!" He mentally called out to Archangel Raphael, who guided him to stop walking and to rub his hands together. As Kevin did so, he clairvoyantly saw sparks of emerald-green light emanating between his fingers. Raphael told him to allow his hand to hover over his pain. Kevin was amazed to see the emerald-green light rush out of his hand into his foot.

When Kevin resumed walking, there was no more pain! He began slowly increasing his pace, and after a few minutes, he was back to his initial speed with no more discomfort. He was able to heal completely thanks to his intuition and the angels.

Gentle Reminders to Move

Many of my (Robert's) clients complain of backache. One thing I teach them, which works miracles, is to set movement reminders on their phone. (After all, it seems that nowadays, people rarely go five seconds separated from their phone; let's use this dependency to our advantage!) Set alarms to go off every two hours. These will be your cues to get up, drink some water, and take a short walk.

It is easy to become so engrossed in your work that you totally lose track of the time. Many have had the experience of working for what seems to be a short period, only to look up and realize it has become dark outside. Time can get away from you when you're in a creative flow. It's important to have an outside force that will protect you and your body. You don't need to move for too long—five minutes is fine. Then you can get back to work. You'll find that your body will thank you by giving you new ideas, inspiration, and enough energy to last two more hours until your next reminder.

When you're home and not working, the alarms don't need to stop! If you tend to zone out on the couch, then please set reminders for these times of the day, too. Sofas have even less support for your sensitive spine than a chair, and can be so terrible for your back. Be sure to gently move around every couple of hours, and you'll notice a difference in your body's state of ease.

Finding the Right Activity for You

Make workouts an activity that you enjoy. Find an exercise or routine that suits your individual needs. You might prefer to work out alone, using just your body weight or free weights. You may find the energy of others motivating, and attempt classes at the gym or other group activities. Think about whether you'd prefer to exercise indoors or engage in an outdoor activity. If you're indoors, what are you looking at—a boring wall or a lovely view of the ocean? All of these things will make a dramatic difference to your experience.

The location of your pain and its severity will determine what activities you can and cannot do. If you are very limited, please speak to your care provider about the safest way to start exercising. It is always best to get professional advice about what is optimal for your body so you do not accidentally do damage. Remember, your goal is a flexible, happy, pain-free body, so it is wise to take the time solicit expert advice.

If you are sedentary, please do not feel that you need to start full steam. An easy walk is more than enough to get your blood flowing. (There's a funny, yet true, saying that applies here: "No matter how slow you're going, you're still running laps around the people on the couch.") As you walk, you're relying on your hips and pelvis to keep you upright. Your muscles activate, and your body corrects itself on a minute scale with each movement. Each step you take is a step closer to a pain-free body.

It is also important not to forget your flexibility. People often focus upon strength training and cardiovascular exercises, overlooking this incredibly important aspect to fitness. When you are tight and inflexible, your muscles are more likely to strain and tear. Stretching loosens the muscle fibers and gives your body a wider range of motion. Try to touch your toes—if you can't, then it shows that your hamstrings are too tight. Engage in gentle stretches, or take a beginning yoga class, to relax your muscles; almost instantly, you will find that you can reach farther.

One of the best ways to alleviate pain is through strengthening your core—your back and abdominal muscles. Time and time again, chronic back pain is linked with poor core strength. If your abdominal muscles are weak, then your spine and pelvis are more inclined to tilt and unbalance. You don't need a six-pack, but internal strength is essential for a happy, pain-free back. The following activities are wonderful ways to start:

— **Tai chi** is a form of exercise from China that involves very gentle movements. It is said that, when done correctly, you are working every muscle within your body. Your moves are slow yet very deliberate, allowing your joints to glide from position to position. Tai chi slowly stretches your muscles, increases your flexibility, and helps improve your balance. Over the years, it has been found to have many health benefits and to help such conditions as arthritis, fatigue, anxiety, pain, poor posture, stress, and tension.

Tai chi is also a lovely spiritual practice with three aspects: health, meditation, and martial arts. Each movement is a sloweddown self-defense technique. Tai chi activates the healing meridians of the body to circulate *chi,* or life force. This creates a flow of potent healing energy that seeks out, and restores function to, areas of imbalance.

— **Yoga** is another wonderful exercise that incorporates spirituality. You learn to connect with your breath and find a sense of oneness while also holding your body in special positions, known as *asanas,* for extended periods of time. Don't worry; you don't need to be a gymnast or contortionist. There are many beginner classes in gyms and studios, as well as books, YouTube videos, and DVDs you can work with at home. Having a yoga teacher ensures that you're safely and correctly performing the stretches. Over time your flexibility will improve, and you'll be able to do deeper and more challenging asanas.

— **Pilates** is a conditioning routine that uses stretches and repetition to increase flexibility, strength, and endurance. It emphasizes muscle control and strengthening your core. Don't be deceived, as the simple-looking exercises are highly effective and can still make you sweat! Some Pilates studios have weighted machines to add an extra dimension to your practice.

The Benefits of Exercise

Even in traumatic, potentially life-threatening accidents, a fit and healthy body is more adapted to cope with pain. Rachel Racklyeft had enjoyed a fulfilling 13-year career as a gym instructor when her life suddenly took a turn on July 25, 2010. That's when this avid horse lover fell from her horse; she knew immediately that she was injured. She also knew, due to her many years of training, that holding still was her best choice.

Rachel was rushed to the hospital, where it was revealed how severely she had been hurt. She had fractured her C7, T1, T2, T3, T4, and T5 vertebrae—from the base of her neck to midway down her back. It was a horrifying discovery, and depressing thoughts rushed through her mind. She wondered, *Will I walk again? Will I ever ride my horse again? Will I ever teach at the gym again?*

Miraculously Rachel still had full sensation in her body. No nerve damage appeared to have taken place! Doctors told her that at some point in the future, she would be able to do the things she loved again. However, to get there, she had to heal not only her spine but also her emotions. Thankfully, Rachel was surrounded by supportive and uplifting people. She discovered who really cared and who her true friends were. The gym told her that her job was secure; everyone just wanted to see her heal.

The days immediately following Rachel's accident were very painful. She was bruised, battered, and emotionally exhausted. The moments she had alone in the hospital, she spent writing in her journal. Not everything she jotted down made sense, but it didn't need to. It was her way of releasing the pressure and pain from inside her head. It was a particular challenge for Rachel to be fitted for a back brace and instructed to wear it for four months. To help herself cope, she named the brace "Bertha."

When she was forced to stop and rest, she took the time to communicate with her angels. She called on them for Divine assistance and prayed for healing. Beautifully, Rachel noticed little signs that let her know her prayers were being heard.

In the months that followed, the pain was terrible, and Rachel found it difficult to get comfortable. She took pharmaceutical pain medication to take the edge off, but was shocked by how quickly the pain came back whenever she tried to reduce her dosage. She found this time to be sad and challenging, because she didn't like being on all those drugs and wished the pain would just go away.

Finally, the time came for "Bertha" to be taken off. It was then that Rachel discovered that her loving family, supportive friends, and guiding angels were her best pain relief. She was able to clear through self-limiting beliefs and let her true self shine through. The more she focused on the things she was grateful for in her life, the more her discomfort decreased. Today Rachel is fully healed and pain-free.

Rachel is able to walk again, ride horses again, and even teach at the gym again. She has a new outlook on life and realizes that when things seem tough, you just have to take it one step at a time. Every year, on the anniversary of her accident, she does something challenging. She pushes herself in new ways to show the universe she is grateful to be alive and wants to experience as much of this life as possible.

Having a balanced mind is necessary—and coupled with a balanced physique, you have a winning combination. Alison Scambary, a fitness instructor for 15 years, knew and understood the importance of a strong and healthy body. For years she had encouraged others to reach their fitness goals, respecting the individual needs of each client. She had a passion for exercise and made it a part of her everyday life, often taking weekend holidays with her husband to challenge themselves with activities such as mountain biking. On one such trip, Alison gained a new perspective on the importance of fitness.

In September 2013, Alison and her husband were biking when she took a bad fall and dislocated her shoulder. The pain was excruciating! Due to her training, she knew that moving her arm would only make matters worse, so she just tried to carefully hold herself in a comfortable position. An ambulance arrived and took her to the hospital, where she unfortunately had to wait with a dislocated shoulder for an exhausting six hours. Alison took some pharmaceutical medication to take the edge off what she described as one of the most painful things she had ever experienced. Once her shoulder was safely back in place, she was free to go home.

Alison discovered that she used her arms for more tasks than she ever realized, further reinforcing for her the importance of a fully functioning, healthy body. Tender shoulder or not, however, she couldn't be kept from exercising! She understood that fitness levels drop rapidly without regular activity, and she didn't want to lose the results of all her hard work. She started with stationary cycling, working at a comfortable pace to avoid pain. Movement helps the body heal from injuries, and the endorphins released during exercise keep moods uplifted. Alison knew that if she became sedentary, it could affect her positive nature—and she wasn't willing to lose that!

When Alison began seeing a physical therapist, the person told her that her recovery time was very impressive; she was healing rapidly and had gained back a great deal of her range and flexibility. The therapist put this down to Alison's commitment to her health and fitness.

With regular exercise, your body becomes more adapted to healing. The tone of your muscles and your core strength accelerate the healing response. You needn't turn into a personal trainer or bodybuilder, but physical fitness can help take your pain away. Release any thoughts that say you can't—give it a try. Start slowly, and you will see the transformation taking place over time.

CHAPTER EIGHT

Physical Therapies and Healing Methods

You can achieve healing in miraculous ways. Sometimes this occurs on its own; other times it involves working with a trusted practitioner who can guide you.

When we evaluate a treatment, we must be aware of its underlying philosophy. Some therapies focus on managing symptoms rather than addressing the true cause. We feel that for a complete healing, you need to address the source. Although symptom alleviation is important, please understand that if you ignore what is creating the problem, it will resurface again and again. Many healers will begin by alleviating your most pressing symptoms. However, as your pain levels decrease, the balance of treatment should change, as your healer puts more focus on the underlying triggers.

In this chapter, we will explain some of the therapies with which we have experience, including those that our clients have given us feedback upon. However, the most important thing to consider when you seek a healing modality for yourself is your own intuition. As you read through the following options, let your Higher Self tell you which would be right for you.

Meditate for a moment on the subheads, even before reading the content. Listen to what your inner voice says before you take in the information. Let this give you ideas for the types of treatment that might be best for you. As you read, you'll get further confirmation on whether it's the right path for you to follow.

Therapeutic Packs for Pain

Too often we reach for a heat pack or hot water bottle for comfort and relief. When the warmth is present, it does make the pain feel better, but is it actually doing anything useful? You'll notice that the pain usually comes back soon after removing the heat. It masks your symptoms rather than healing the situation. Let's investigate why.

Heat can attract more heat. When you remove the source of the warmth, the surface cools down rapidly, but the heat can remain trapped within the area. This creates inflammation, and then the pain returns. The sudden temperature change can also shock the muscles and trigger a spasm.

A similar process happens with ice packs, in which the cold causes your vessels to constrict, pushing blood away from the area. This can be a valuable resource for acute injuries, because you don't want to give the inflammation a chance to take hold. Using a cold pack often, however, such as you would with a chronic injury, will severely restrict the circulation in the area. Once the ice is removed, the blood rushes back in and pools there, leading to heat and inflammation. So, while you may find initial relief, the pain quickly reappears when you take away the ice pack.

A more balanced solution than either a hot or ice pack is a *cool* pack. This involves placing a wheat pack, which is commonly heated in the microwave, in the fridge instead. It must stay there for a minimum of four hours to adequately chill. Then you can remove the pack from the fridge and apply it to your area of discomfort. You will instantly feel a cool sensation, and your muscles will relax as tension is released. Then, when you remove the cool pack, the pain stays away.

You can also use the healing power of the earth by making a warm sea-salt pack. Simply place one cup of fine-grain Celtic, Atlantic, Himalayan, or Dead Sea salt into a bowl. (If you purchase coarse salt, just crush it up a little in your blender first.) Next, pour in a tablespoon of boiling water, and mix the salt around until everything is just moistened. The mixture should stay together when you take a handful, but be moist enough that you can still feel some warmth.

Sit or lie in a comfortable position, and place a good amount of the salt on the afflicted area. If the grains refuse to stay in place, you can bandage them into position. As the warmth enters your skin, your muscles will relax. Minute amounts of the salt will be absorbed by your skin, giving you micronutrients that help release inflammation. Leave the salt in place for up to one hour. When you're finished, you can discard the salt and have a warm shower or bath.

For additional anti-inflammatory benefits, add 10 drops of peppermint essential oil to the salt. If you notice any skin irritations (either with or without the peppermint oil), discontinue use and consult a health-care professional.

Essential Oils That Heal Pain

Essential oils are concentrates from flowers, leaves, seeds, bark, or fruits of different plants. They are potent remedies for healing and have both a physical and spiritual application. In addition, each oil transcends the physical world and combines with your energy for a truly powerful healing. While each will treat a number of physical complaints, in this book we focus on their applications in pain relief.

Essential oils haven't often been studied for their ability to heal pain. However, some researchers are looking at the use of aromatherapy as an adjunct to conventional medical treatment. While there are suggestions that essential oils can enhance the effects of other treatments, many say that the relaxation qualities alone are enough to help someone with chronic pain. When the mind is relaxed, our perception of pain is different. The more we relax and let go, the less we focus on chronic pain.

A little *is* known about the compounds in each oil. We must consider the thousands of case studies from practitioners that show a definite improvement when using essential oils. These potent plant remedies heal.

The major issue when using essential oils is quality. You must find high-quality brands to get a good result. Unfortunately, there are many essential oils on the market that are diluted or, even worse, synthetic. Look for 100 percent pure essential oils. Sometimes more expensive oils, such as rose, will be diluted in jojoba oil. This is perfectly fine as long as you're aware of it. Be cautious, as some brands do not clearly label their products, and you won't be sure if the contents are pure.

The more expensive oils are often the better-quality ones. However, please don't rush out and buy the priciest bottles you can find without doing your research on the manufacturer first. It would also be wise to avoid companies that rely on multilevel marketing strategies, as the energy impacts the quality of the oil.

The following oils are the most common ones used for pain relief.

Peppermint

Peppermint oil naturally contains menthol, which is the active ingredient in many topical gels and sprays for pain relief because of its localized anesthetic properties. Peppermint oil causes blood vessels to dilate, so you may get some initial redness as it kicks in. Afterward, your circulation will improve and helpful cells will be able to repair any damage, which can trigger a cascade of healing reactions.

Try peppermint oil for sore muscles, joints, and backs. Apply 3 drops to an organic cotton ball, and rub onto the tender area. If you experience excessive skin irritation, discontinue use immediately and wipe away with a warm, wet cloth.

In 2002, *The Clinical Journal of Pain* published a study in which peppermint oil was used to treat nerve pain. In this case, a 76-year-old woman had terrible nerve pain after a viral infection. Standard treatments were not working, so the physicians tried peppermint oil. The patient was instructed to apply neat (or straight) peppermint oil onto the affected areas. She noticed almost immediate relief, and they found the analgesic action lasted 4 to 6 hours. Two months later, she was still using the oil and had only very minor side effects. This led the team to consider further research into the uses of peppermint oil.

Lavender

Lavender oil is well known for its ability to calm and relax. Many people will inhale this familiar fragrance to help with sleep or to soothe anxiety. However, lavender oil is also excellent at relaxing muscles. The more your mind is quieted, the less angry your body feels. This is why healing your physical pain requires that we also pay attention to your mind.

Lavender oil clears your third-eye chakra, awakening your spiritual sight. It helps you to be simultaneously strong and sensitive. You'll be aware of energies, feelings, and sensations, but they won't overwhelm you. Instead you will be in control of the situation.

You hold the key to your successful outcome. Deep down you know the solution to your problem. Often, it's simply a matter of releasing. Lavender helps you to let go. Its scent relaxes your mind *and* your muscles. Applying a few drops to your neck and shoulders will penetrate the tension and release muscle aches as the aroma touches your soul and balances your mind. The angels say it's like watching an ice cube melt—what was once hard and unyielding transforms into a free-flowing, flexible state.

Apply a drop or two of lavender oil to your temples to ease a headache. It's particularly good for tension headaches, but will heal any kind. Gently massage the oil into your temples and around the back of your neck, right up to the occiput (the area where your neck muscles attach to your skull). Within minutes, your headache will disappear.

Chamomile

There are two types of chamomile: Roman and German. We prefer the use of German chamomile because it's been more widely researched and has a healing vibration.

The oil of German chamomile is blue, which is connected with the throat chakra. This is your center of communication and speaking your truth. You needn't be afraid of speaking up. The angels give you messages that they want you to convey. It can be frightening to speak to others about sensitive topics. But if you're being urged to do so, healing will take place. Perhaps part of your purpose is to show people a different view, or maybe you will say the perfect words to comfort a situation. You won't know until you speak up. Always trust that these thoughts and feeling are coming from your Higher Self and the angels. You're being given the gift of clear communication!

Chamomile eases inflammation, pain, and tension. Azulene, the compound that gives the oil its distinctive color, has anti-inflammatory and skin-healing properties. However, like all plant medicines, no single chemical is doing all the work. All the parts work in unison to create a wonderfully balanced healing symphony.

Apply three or four drops of German chamomile to the area of discomfort. If you get a little on your hands, take a moment to inhale the fragrance. The aroma transcends the physical and uplifts your soul. Let yourself have that moment of painlessness.

Wintergreen

This oil has a high concentration of methyl salicylate, which contains the same component that gives aspirin its pain-relieving effect. Many people have found success with this oil. However, in our experience, wintergreen is often too overpowering for sensitive people. It can cause skin irritation, so if you feel guided to try this oil, please do so carefully. Apply it to a small test area first, and notice what effects it might have immediately, then a day later.

Ways to Work with Healing Oils

All of the oils mentioned here can be safely applied directly to the skin. Some oils, however, are meant to be used only through certain methods, so always consult the directions or a qualified professional. If you notice any irritation, even with an oil that you have used successfully before, discontinue use and wipe the area clean.

Diffusers

You might want to invest in an aromatherapy diffuser, which will send tiny molecules of these healing oils into the air. As you inhale the fragrance, your mind and body will be uplifted. You can start the diffuser when you get home after a busy day, and allow yourself to unwind. Remember that relaxation is a very important key in your pain-free life.

Carriers

A carrier dilutes essential oils to make them more tolerable to your skin. With pure oils, a little goes a long way. You can add 40 drops of any essential oil to 1 ounce (30 ml/2 tablespoons) of a neutral oil such as organic coconut or olive oil.

Coconut oil is solid at room temperature, so to make a sooth-ing rub, warm 2 tablespoons in a small saucepan on the lowest possible heat. Once melted, add 40 drops of your desired essential oils, then pour the mixture into a small, heatproof jar. Glass jars work well for this, and you can often purchase small jars from your health-food store. After the oil has cooled and set into a semisolid, cap it tightly. Then, whenever you need it, take a small amount of the ointment and gently massage it into the painful area. A little will go a long way, because the solid oil melts once it warms to your body temperature. If there is little improvement after a few days, you can add more essential oils by melting your batch again.

To make our favorite Pain-Relieving Coconut Rub, follow the above instructions with 1 tablespoon of organic coconut oil, 20 drops peppermint oil, 15 drops lavender oil, and 10 drops German chamomile oil.

Soothing Relaxation Baths

An aromatherapy bath spreads the inviting scent of the oils through the room and allows small concentrations to be absorbed into your skin. You'll step out of the bath feeling wonderfully comfortable, relaxed, and happy.

Since oil and water don't mix, we can't just sprinkle oil in the bathtub. Instead, add 15 drops of essential oils into a cup of organic apple cider vinegar. The vinegar will help dissolve the oils, as well as add its own healing benefits for your body. You may also be guided to include some natural sea salts to the water to further purify your energy and soothe your muscles. Natural sea salt contains a variety of healing microminerals, such as magnesium. Epsom salts can also be like a therapeutic massage for sore muscles.

For a healing experience, sprinkle ½ cup natural sea salt and ½ cup Epsom salts into your bathwater. Mix 2 drops of peppermint, 10 drops of chamomile, and 3 drops of lavender oil to 1 cup of or-ganic apple cider vinegar, then add to your bath. Stir until every-thing is dissolved, then sit back and relax. You'll feel the tension leaving your body within 15 minutes. Take a moment to visualize your body releasing its pain. See it as a dark energy being drawn out into the water, with no way for it to return. When you pull the plug to drain the water, reaffirm the release of your pain.

Manual Therapies to Heal Pain

A 2013 study investigated the prevalence of pain in Australians. For those who saw a doctor, 19.2 percent suffered from chronic pain, most commonly osteoarthritis and backaches. More than 86 percent of patients used medication for it, and one-third were also seeking nonpharmaceutical methods of relief.

Natural therapies and alternative medicines are excellent remedies for pain. There are some interventions that aren't completely understood by modern science; however, the simple fact is that they work. Those who try them commonly report a reduction in their discomfort and inflammation. Even though we may not fully understand the mechanisms, it would be ignorant to dismiss these modalities entirely.

Some therapies have gotten a bad rap over the years, but many are very powerful when done correctly. However, it is usually the rare, unfortunate experiences that get public attention. Sadly, the media focuses on negativity, showing us horrible things happening around the world and casting many healers in an unfavorable light. Yet the majority of people are wonderful and passionate, and intend nothing but good for others.

Whenever you see a story about a fraudulent healer, always check the story further. You'll often find that the person wasn't a qualified member of his or her alleged profession at all. This is why it is so important to always check the credentials of your therapists. Professional healing associations require that their members adhere to certain ethical standards. Often, they also mandate a certain amount of continuing professional education so therapists can apply new skills and the most up-to-date information in their practice.

The following are some of the best therapies to incorporate into your path toward wellness.

Massage

During a massage, a therapist warms your muscles and releases tension from your body. It is easy to feel at peace and surrender to the moment. This can be an excellent method for soothing tension, back pain, and neck and shoulder complaints. When deciding which style to try, keep in mind that each was designed for a different purpose. Two of the most common are *Swedish* and *remedial*.

— **Swedish massage** is wonderfully relaxing. It uses a reasonable amount of pressure, just enough so that the muscles respond. The therapist applies flowing, rhythmic movements, allowing both your body and mind to release stress and tension. You can let go and melt into the healing table.

The angels describe Swedish massage as like an aura dance. Practitioners work with your energy as much as they work with your physical body, so it's important to have a happy, high-energy therapist. You don't need someone sending anger or negativity into you.

— **Remedial massage**, such as deep-tissue massage, is usually what people ask for when they're in pain. It is important to note that it may initially cause even more discomfort. Therapists use firm pressure and focus on isolating specific muscles rather than being concerned with general relaxation, as in a Swedish massage. They begin by warming the surrounding tissues, then follow their fingers to the site of your pain, concentrating on the muscle causing the problem. They target the trigger points that run through each muscle, allowing it to release. Given that they are massaging the specific area of pain, you can be very uncomfortable until your body lets go.

I (Robert) learned Swedish and remedial massage as part of my naturopathy degree, which gave me insight into both these therapies. As part of training, we had to complete quite a few hours of practical clinic work in which a supervisor monitored us as we worked on clients. Clients would come in and describe their complaint, then we would get to it.

At this point, I'd been working on my spirituality for many years and had learned how to tune in to the body. I discovered that I could feel when clients' muscles released their tension, which was usually after 15 to 20 minutes of work. Unfortunately, I was expected to keep massaging for the remainder of the hour-long appointment, and as I continued, I could feel the areas under my fingers getting irritated again. By the end of the session, those poor muscles were tense again. I conveyed this feeling to my supervisors, but they didn't heed my warnings.

It is easy to cause yourself more harm if you ignore the signals given by your body. An hour-long massage can be a luxurious treat, but only when the work is balanced. We feel that the two styles work best together—remedial massage until the muscle releases, then gentle, rhythmic Swedish strokes through the rest of the body.

This is why it is important to research your massage practitioner first and ask if he or she works on an intuitive level. You may be surprised to find that many popular therapists are highly spiritual. Some might keep this a secret in order to not deter potential clients, but they will soon come to understand that their spirituality is the precise reason you're being guided to them. Also ask if they use aromatherapy during the massage. This is a nice bonus, as it gets your senses going on a physical, emotional, and spiritual level. Your body lets go of tension as you inhale the delicate perfume from the healing essential oils. Some practitioners will create custom blends for your particular needs.

Bowen Therapy

Developed in Australia, Bowen therapy is a subtle, noninvasive, therapeutic form of bodywork that has gained popularity all around the world. It began with Tom Bowen's work on people with pain. He would apply gentle pressure or a small rolling movement at specific areas, following his intuitive guidance. Most patients felt almost immediate relief! Word spread, and people traveled great distances to see him. He reported seeing 280 patients per week in 1973, and in 1976 he treated approximately 13,000 patients. These astonishing numbers are the perfect testament to Bowen's intuitive guidance, showing that he was healing at a deep level. After many years of successful practice, he began to teach his methods, and after his passing in 1982, his technique lived on as Bowen therapy.

During a Bowen treatment, your therapist will ensure that you feel relaxed and safe before beginning to apply a sequence of slight movements at specific areas of your body. These manipulations trigger healing reactions; an adjustment at one point causes the vibration to move through the entire length of the muscle, rather like flicking the string on a guitar. This is why a practitioner often works on areas other than where you feel the pain.

An unusual aspect of a Bowen treatment is that therapists will engage in a short pause between movements, which allows your body to really absorb the messages that they have sent through. It is best not to overload your system with too many messages at once, and this break allows practitioners to see how your body responds to each slight adjustment. Then they can assess what move to make next, or whether the body should be allowed to continuing balancing itself a little longer.

Bowen therapy corrects physical imbalances and utilizes muscle memory to bring your body back to harmony. It starts a cascade of healing responses that continue working up to 48 hours later. So while you may not notice anything immediately after a session, you will soon after. Clients often feel some improvement right away, then continue feeling better and better as the day continues.

Only four or five treatments are needed in many cases, and some complaints are healed after a single session.

Ask practitioners how they work before you make your appointment. Some will leave the room momentarily, to give your body privacy as it triggers the reactions it needs. Intuitive therapists will often want to stay in the room with you, and some will speak with you during treatment to help you release stored emotions or stress. While there used to be a strict rule of not including other therapies while using Bowen, this policy is being phased out as many discover the benefits of adding other modalities. Some Bowen practitioners will now incorporate energy methods during their pauses to activate your body's innate ability to heal itself.

If you choose to use other therapies alongside Bowen, ensure that you do so in the correct order. Since this is a subtle technique, more heavy-handed therapies can undo its work. Just be sure to have your chiropractic work, physiotherapy, or massages done a day or two *before* your Bowen session in order to reap the greatest benefits from all of them!

Physiotherapy

Physiotherapy, also known simply as physical therapy, can involve stretches, exercises, and rehabilitation techniques. A physiotherapist (or physical therapist) will isolate the muscles that are causing you pain, working with your body to get your range of motion back to what it should be. Sometimes therapists engage in assisted stretching, in which they take your muscle to the point of restriction, then gently push it to go a little further. This can cause some discomfort initially, but when done correctly, it can grant you greater flexibility. Some will also work with ultrasound machines to heal muscles on a deeper level, sending waves of energy into your body and triggering it to repair.

Physiotherapists know the muscles of the body very well. They are able to assess your complaint and explain which parts are causing the problem. If you are sensitive, explain this to your therapist, and request that they start with gentler approaches. Once you feel more comfortable, you will have no problem completing the stretches they recommend.

Chiropractic

A chiropractor addresses structural imbalances within the spine, using manual manipulations to adjust your vertebrae. If you've had long-term issues, you may require frequent sessions. It is important to ask your chiropractor what might be causing the situation and if there is anything you can adapt in your everyday life for better comfort. Knowledge of your body and its triggers can be an incredibly powerful tool.

Some chiropractors focus on superficial relief and maintenance rather than treating the underlying cause of your discomfort. Work with a practitioner who individualizes your visits. If someone does the same thing to each patient every time, and says to come back in two weeks, consider a different therapist. You want someone whose focus is on healing work rather than getting more clients and booking more appointments.

The thought of someone making forceful movements to your spine can be frightening, so remember to always check your therapist's credentials first. A practitioner who continues his or her education, attending seminars and training days every year, will be a great asset to your health.

Acupuncture

The healing method of acupuncture is thousands of years old and comes from traditional Chinese medicine. It is based on the idea that there are energy channels, or *meridians,* that run through the body and connect our *chakras,* our energy centers. When our chakras are clear, we can circulate energy, but the energy flows differently if there are imbalances or blocks. Traditional Chinese medicine says that those blockages can cause pain and other health issues. Consider water: without movement, it is stagnant and unhealthy, but flowing water is an essential component of life.

Acupuncturists have identified very specific areas on the body that act as release points. When influenced, these points open up the floodgates of energy and allow the body to heal itself. Tiny needles are inserted at those points and left for a time, usually from 15 minutes up to one hour. Even those worried about needles usually say that acupuncture isn't frightening—the benefits outweigh the phobia. However, be certain that your practitioner takes proper sanitary measures. He or she should *never* reuse needles and must dispose of them in a proper container.

Modern research has found that acupuncture does work, although scientists are not quite sure of the reasons why, as they do not give weight to the knowledge of traditional Chinese medicine. However, perhaps it's not essential to understand how it works when the results speak for themselves. We ask you to question friends and family who have undergone acupuncture treatments. You'll find that most of them had positive results.

For example, I (Robert) have never been very good at treating heel spurs. I work with patients to alleviate the discomfort, but it's usually temporary. Unless the spur is dissolved or removed surgically, the pain keeps coming back. There are some naturopathic herbal medicines that can, in theory, dissolve the heel spurs, but it's a very lengthy process. That being said, I've referred several patients to acupuncturists, and they received lasting improvement after just a couple of sessions. Now they can walk pain-free.

One lady healed her stomach pain by listening to her guidance and trying acupuncture. In an attempt to treat her acne, she received a prescription medication that would also alter her hormones. It worked well for the first month, but then gave her terrible side effects. She was waking up every day feeling depressed and tired. She had such bad stomach pain that it stopped her from eating. She spent many emotional hours in tears.

She called her doctor to make an appointment, but something inside her knew she needed to look at alternative options. She took some time to meditate and got a strong feeling that her angels wanted her to try something different. She was guided to a friend who knew a lot about Chinese medicine. This person recommended a practitioner, who suggested that she try acupuncture. After her first session, she felt amazing! She had more energy, and the stomach pain was gone. This woman continued following the guidance of her angels and her traditional Chinese medicine practitioner, and today she is happy, healthy, and pain-free.

Find the Perfect Practitioner for You

You will be sensitive to the energy of your healing practitioner. Ask your angels to guide you to the perfect person by saying:

"Dear God and angels, please show me clear signs that I can easily understand and interpret to indicate who is the right practitioner for me. I ask that they be happy, compassionate, and walk their talk. I trust your Divine decision and know you will send the perfect person for me. Thank you."

Many readers have shared how they were miraculously directed to the right therapist by saying a prayer similar to this. When you work with intuitive practitioners, they can share alternative ideas that you might not have looked into. As you let the angels guide you, your healing will begin.

⁓

Many people have experienced healing visitations by someone who mysteriously vanishes after coming to the rescue. Tiina Agur, an Estonian woman who works in Luxembourg, had been suffering from hip pain when an angel guided her through the replacement surgery.

Her surgery was in 2013 (on the ninth day of the ninth month at 9 A.M.). She felt comfortable and relaxed as she was being wheeled to the operating room. The staff had wrapped her in green sheets that kept her warm and content.

A woman who looked to be about 65 appeared by her bedside. She was wearing surgical scrubs and some kind of hair covering. She looked faintly Nordic in her appearance: bright blue eyes; tanned, as if from spending most of her time outdoors; lots of wrinkles; and the kindest, most comforting smile. She took Tiina's hand in both of hers and held it, smiling, as she said, "Hello. I am your anesthetist."

Tiina thought it was very, very kind of her to take a moment to reassure her in such a way. After that, she doesn't remember a thing. Her last thought was how peaceful she felt with this gentle woman watching over her.

The next day Tiina was swapping stories with her hospital roommate. She expressed to her how lovely the older lady was and wondered whether her roommate had the same anesthetist. She said no, hers had been a young man. Still curious, Tiina proceeded to ask several nurses if they knew the anesthetist. All of them said that there was no such person. And, shaking their heads, they said that Tiina had probably dreamed it all.

Tiina knows it wasn't a dream; her anesthetist had been an angel. Now she is getting used to her new hip. When she feels discomfort, she thinks of her anesthetist's kind face and it makes her feel better.

೧

Karen Malone had a lifelong dream to become a flight attendant. She achieved her goal and marveled at the miracle of flight every single time the aircraft took off. She would affectionately refer to the plane as her "office." Little did she know that she'd meet the answer to her prayers on board.

A short time before that fateful flight, Karen had endured the loss of her beloved mother and the breakdown of her marriage. These emotional traumas happened within weeks of one another. Karen also suffered from agonizing back pain. She saw her doctor, but after a battery of tests, nothing was found to explain it. She tried a number of prescriptions from her back specialist, but her pain seemed to worsen.

During this time, Karen connected to her spirituality. She began asking her angels for help and welcomed them into her life. Some days it was a struggle to get dressed and make it to work, but she persisted. She feared what the future might hold, as she never wanted to give up the joy of flying.

One evening, as Karen was serving drinks on a red-eye flight across America, a very distinguished-looking passenger asked her, "What's wrong with your hips?" As a flight attendant, Karen had heard it all. She brushed this off as just another bizarre question, among the many directed at her. She politely thanked him for his concern and told him that it was her back that was giving her problems. Not satisfied with her reply, the passenger insisted she had hip problems. He explained he would come visit her after the flight. Previous passengers had told Karen about every miracle cure known, so she braced herself for another sales pitch. As it happened, her interaction with this man would change her life forever.

The gentleman was a retired doctor. He explained that his own discomfort had led to his early retirement. He handed Karen a scrap of paper with a nurse's name on it and insisted she call to set up an appointment immediately. He told her that there was a team of specialists in Atlanta, and she should tell them he'd sent her. His parting words as he deplaned were, "These people will give you back your life."

Could this be real? Karen wondered. Was it possible that God had arranged for this man to be on the same flight as she was to help her heal? She kept the piece of paper but didn't follow the doctor's orders right away. Instead, she persisted with another round of painful spinal injections that gave her little relief. One day, hardly able to walk, Karen found that paper and made the call. She had exhausted all other options and wanted to investigate this further. Even as she left a message, she was still in disbelief. She left a rambling message saying that if they believe in angels, this man was on board her flight and said to call.

Fifteen minutes later a nurse called back and replied, "Yes, I believe in angels, and we love the doctor who referred you. How can we help you?" Tears of joy streamed down Karen's face as she told her story. The nurse assured Karen that she would get treatment within the next few months. Karen explained she couldn't handle the pain for that length of time. The nurse felt for her, and fit her in two days later when there was a cancellation.

Karen was put under the excellent care of a young doctor and had a successful hip replacement surgery. Then, just two short months later, she had another. When she awoke from her second surgery, the doctor was seated beside her. He said, "Today we gave you back your life." At first, Karen wondered if she had died on the operating table. Then the doctor explained that he'd found a large bone spur on her hip. It was affecting the joint and creating a hole through the hip bone. If it hadn't been found, Karen would have been in a wheelchair for the rest of her life.

Her angels brought Karen the healing referral she needed 30,000 feet in the air! Six weeks later, she was back at work: pain-free, comfortable, and standing tall.

Trust Your Guidance

Sometimes the guidance we receive might not make total sense. Rather than judging it, explore it to see what occurs. My (Doreen's) husband, Michael, was having horrible migraines, which became more severe during solar flares. Being so sensitive, he could not tolerate over-the-counter drugs—nor did he want to!—so he first tried several natural approaches. Nothing made a difference. Michael and I asked Robert for his advice, and he prescribed the herbal medicine *Ginkgo biloba*. This herb enhances the circulation in the head and helps relieve the pressure. It took the edge off, but Michael still felt a great deal of pain.

Michael went within and asked his body what it needed. He received the guidance that his body was like a battery, or electrical circuit. He saw that drinking apple cider vinegar with honey would help to alkalize his body and allow the battery to recharge.

It worked! He now drinks vinegar two or three times a day and hasn't had a headache since.

❧

Rachael White sought help from conventional medicine, but ultimately followed her inner guidance to heal her son's pain. He'd had severe eczema since he was five, and it was continually getting worse. He was sent home from school one day because his skin was broken and bleeding, which administrators said posed a health risk to others. He was kept from playing sports, and children teased him about his skin. The eczema also prevented him from swimming in the ocean because the saltwater stung his wounds.

Rachael asked her local doctor for help, but was devastated when he said, "I'm sorry, but there's nothing I can do for your son." She then rushed to make an appointment with a specialist, who told her to bathe her son in bleach! The specialist said that this would kill any bacterial infection and give the skin time to heal. Rachael politely declined and said she would explore alternative options before trying something that seemed so drastic.

It was then that Rachael pursued her spiritual path. Her angels guided her to use a combination of essential oils, nutrition, and meditation to help her son. He is now nine years old, and he no longer has eczema!

❧ ❧

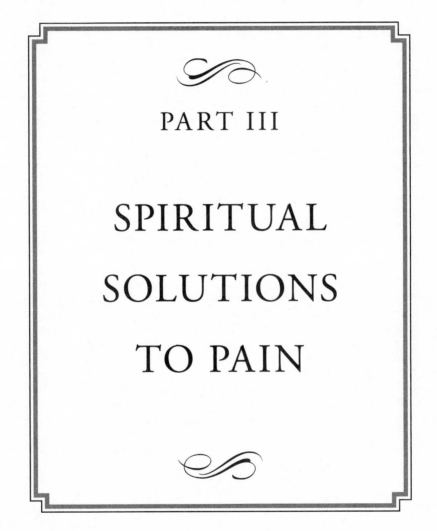

PART III

SPIRITUAL SOLUTIONS TO PAIN

CHAPTER NINE

ENERGETICALLY EVICTING PAIN

Negative energy is the home of suffering. The more you take on, the more susceptible you become to its effects. It perpetuates itself in an unhealthy cycle—the more pain you feel, the more negative energy you attract. But when you clear away the darkness, you can feel the loving presence of your angels. You'll remember that in spiritual truth, you're already perfect, whole, and complete. It's merely an illusion of pain that's holding you down.

Let's evict the hurt from your beautiful body with some energetic healing methods, so that only pure health can remain.

Connecting with Nature

Mother Nature is a beautiful healer. A lot of the hurts we accumulate can be partly due to the fact that so many of us live and work indoors. It isn't natural for any creature, including humans. We aren't meant to breathe air-conditioned air or work under artificial lighting. In fact, studies show that many modern illnesses came into being precisely at the time that artificial lighting became commonplace!

We need sunlight in moderation to trigger the brain's production of the feel-good chemical serotonin. Serotonin is also the precursor to melatonin, which the body needs in order to sleep and repair itself. Serotonin regulates the pain response and can reduce its severity. Without enough production of these chemicals, we wake up feeling tired, achy, grumpy, and hungry for junk food.

We also need sunlight to ensure that we're getting adequate vitamin D in our system. While you never want to get sunburned, avoiding the sun too much is also dangerous. The angels say that full-spectrum lighting is necessary for optimal health; the rainbow prism within sunlight feeds each of the colors within the chakra system, as it's also a rainbow. For example, if you're having stomach complaints or power struggles, the yellow within the full-spectrum light would support their healing, because yellow is the color of the solar-plexus chakra, which is associated with these issues.

Please read the ingredients list on sunblock carefully before applying it. Many of these products are loaded with toxic chemicals. The pores on your skin are like tiny mouths drinking in the lotions you apply. Always be sure to choose organic sunscreens, available at your local health-food store or online.

In addition, the angels say that moonlight, starlight, sunsets, and sunrises also increase our overall wellness and heal our pain:

- *Sunrise:* Watching a sunrise awakens the chakras, providing a natural boost of energy. This vitality helps us accomplish our goals for the day with positivity and motivation.

- *Sunset:* Gazing at a sunset helps our chakras relax, and prepares us for a good night's sleep. It cleanses us from the day's activities and allows pain to be dissolved.

- *Starlight:* Being outside beneath the stars triggers our creativity, and helps us be more artistic. Here is where we get the inspiration to overcome pain. We may get thoughts of new treatments we had not considered, and be guided to the perfect practitioner.

- *Moonlight:* Since ancient times, our ancestors have stood beneath the full moon as a powerful method of releasing everything that's toxic from their lives.

Crystal Therapy

Crystals are healing stones that carry an inherent energy. As your spiritual gifts awaken, you will feel a gentle pulse of energy when you hold one. They store and direct healing energies, which your body can easily absorb. When you sit with a crystal and set your intentions, it gives the stone a way to direct its power.

The following are some wonderful crystals and stones for healing pain:

- *Amethyst* transforms the low energy of fear into love. It heightens your intuition so you will know the right way to move forward.

- *Black onyx* pulls out old pain and expectations of pain from your body.

- *Blue lace agate* clears anxiety and stress, bringing comfort to your nerves.

- *Rose quartz* opens your heart and lets peace settle in. Everything that comes from a place of love is healing.

Others crystals that may bring you relief include garnets, clear quartz, ametrine, carnelian, red jasper, sodalite, fluorite, and tiger's eye. Wear, hold, work, or sleep next to these crystals to receive their healing support. (In the Appendix, we recommend certain crystals for particular ailments.)

Cleansing Your Crystals

Crystals are sensitive tools that can easily absorb negative energies; therefore, it's best to cleanse your crystals the first time you bring them home. This is a nice little treat for your crystals, and shows that you appreciate them. It also removes all past associations—the energies of previous owners, countries, and environments—leaving behind pure healing energy. Crystals come from all over the planet and must endure being lifted from the earth, sorted by miners, packed by wholesalers, priced by retailers, and fondled by customers, before finally making their way to you. They can be depleted and drained from their long journey.

Also, be sure to cleanse your crystals if you haven't done so for some time. Think of how many times you walk past them every day. Crystals are like sponges. Since they want to help, they continually clear heavy and lower energies from you. This is a lovely service that they are doing for you. Cleansing them regularly is your way of repaying them for the healing they've been giving unbeknownst to you.

There are a number of ways to cleanse your crystals. Choose a method that feels right for you. A common practice is to bathe the stone in a bowl of saltwater; however, we don't recommend this because the salt can damage the surface of polished stones and may cause clusters to break apart. Try one of the following safer methods:

- Bury the crystal in a bowl of uncooked brown rice. Leave it overnight, then discard the rice in the morning.

- Bury the crystal in a bowl of fresh flower petals; it will be energized and cleansed.

- Light a stick of your favorite incense, and pass the crystal through the smoke. As you light the incense, set the intention that the smoke will clear away all negative vibrations. Imagine a pure white light coming from the incense and awakening the healing properties of your crystal.

Archangel Michael is excellent at clearing negative energies from your crystals. Call upon him by saying:

"Archangel Michael, I ask you to send your purifying energy into my healing crystals. Please awaken their inner knowledge to heal and inspire. Please prepare my crystals for healing work and align them with my energy now. Thank you."

Programming Your Crystals

After cleansing your crystals, be sure to charge them with positive energy. You can do so through prayer: open your heart and express your gratitude to them. You can also leave your stones in sun- or moonlight for four hours.

Now your crystals are ready to be programmed with your loving thoughts. It is important to work *with* the crystals—don't just tell them what to do. Speak to the stones as if they're loving friends, which they are. Pour your heart out and admit any concerns or fears. Let the crystals know exactly what you hope for. Also, share your previous experiences. Include in your prayer that you're willing to accept whatever God and the angels may bring. If they see an easier method for success, be open to it! It is not necessary to use any special words or phrases to program your crystals; it's all about your intention. When your intention is pure, you'll receive the best possible outcome.

Have the courage to step out of your comfort zone and speak from your heart. It might feel strange to talk to a stone, but try explaining your situation to them as if speaking to a compassionate friend. You have nothing to lose by doing this—except the sensation of pain!

Crystal Elixir

Crystals have a healing aura that can be infused into liquids. Many healers simply add stones to their drinking water; while this is fine with some forms of quartz, there are many minerals and crystals that are harmful in water. For example, selenite may dissolve completely. It is also difficult to properly eliminate dust and germs from the surface of the object, and you don't want to be drinking an elixir of bacteria!

The angels have shown us a safe and easy way to work with the energy of crystals. Crystal energy easily passes through glass into the water. So all you need to do is pour water into a clean container, then surround the exterior base with your chosen healing crystals. You'll receive the energy without the fear of contamination.

Choose crystals that will heal pain, such as amethyst, black onyx, blue lace agate, and rose quartz. Rose quartz, in particular, brings a very gentle, calming, and heart-opening energy to your water.

You can arrange the crystals in the evening before bed, and wake up to a crystal-infused elixir.

The Power of the Moon

The cycle of the moon is one of life's constants. You can be sure that it will grow to full and wane into a sliver, and then the cycle repeats. By aligning with the energy of this rhythm, you can choose the perfect time to pray for your goals, whether relating to health or otherwise.

Many religious and spiritual practices are tied into the moon cycles, such as Easter.

As the moon goes from new to full, also known as *growing* or *waxing,* it's the perfect time to pray for things you'd like to attract. It's an opportunity to ask for healing, abundance, like-minded friends, and the opening of new doors.

As the moon goes from full to new, also known as *fading* or *waning,* it's the ideal time to release. Let go of toxins, pain, heartache, and dis-ease. By working with this simple universal truth, you can add an extra dimension of strength to your prayers.

In truth there is nothing more influential than prayer. You're harnessing the power of the Divine and allowing all your angels to intervene for your highest good. When you ask for heavenly assistance, your needs will always be served.

At times you may ignore or simply not notice the guidance that Heaven is trying to give to you. Thankfully, your angels never become annoyed, frustrated, or angry. They love you unconditionally and continue to send you important messages until you understand them. They know that you're human—even though you're a spiritual being in truth, you're still on Earth having a human experience. This means you're prone to mistakes and can easily get caught up in the everyday activities of life. Rest assured that your angels never leave your side—not even for a second. They are with you, guiding you every step of the way.

Following is a full-moon ceremony you might wish to partake in. Feel free to modify it to suit yourself and allow your intuition to guide the entire process.

Full-Moon Release

Supplies:
white candle
pen
sheet of paper
amethyst crystal

Prepare yourself for the full-moon ceremony by relaxing and being willing to let go. You might choose to take a bath or shower to cleanse yourself.

Carry your supplies outside, and situate yourself in an area where you won't be disturbed. Stand or sit under the full moon. It's okay if clouds cover the light; the energy of the celestial sphere will still come through strongly.

Hold the unlit white candle up to the moon and say:

"Please shine your light to all places, seen and unseen. I ask the light to illuminate my aura to remind me of my true state of health. I am willing to release all that no longer serves me and all that has caused me pain in the past. It's time to move on. Angels, please support me in this healing as I cleanse from all that is unbalanced. Thank you."

Light the candle and take a moment to gaze upon the flame. Light travels from the moon to the candle, and from the flame to your heart. Allow the warmth to soften your emotions and give you the courage to let go.

Pick up the pen and at the top of your sheet of paper write: *I am willing to let go and release.* Then list all that you no longer need. Consider such things as: pain, discomfort, heartache, anger, resentment, jealousy, unforgiveness, confusion, and doubt.

Take hold of the amethyst, lift it up to the moon, and say:

"Amethyst, please transform all these negative thoughts and feelings into high energy, happiness, and health."

Wrap the paper around the crystal, or fold it up and place the amethyst on top. Set it in a place where you'll see it regularly, but not constantly. Atop a bedroom dresser or a shelf in the study is a good location.

In one month, open up the paper. Read all the things that you wanted to release, and check off those that are now gone. Then throw away the paper.

If you like, you can repeat this ceremony for the new month ahead.

Full-Moon Water Blessing

The angels have guided us to enhance the energy of the water we drink. Through this ritual, you too can be drinking in the vitality and vibration of love.

Gabriel and the other angels suggest that you place drinking water under the light of the full moon, whose energy is intense with manifestation. Archangel Gabriel says that you can use glass-bottled water purchased from the store, or you can make a special healing batch to enjoy for several days. Allow the water to rest overnight, covered to prevent contamination.

We've found that moon-blessed water tastes sweeter and has a palpable vibration. Drinking it aids you in letting go of the things that no longer serve you and in welcoming fresh energy for your next phase in life.

Tree Therapy

Trees are powerful healers and teachers for those who are sensitive enough to hear their voices. I (Doreen) sat beneath trees and wrote about their messages in my book *Healing with the Fairies*. I find that each tree (like people) has a specific life purpose. Some will help you boost your confidence, others help with relationship issues, some help manifest abundance, and so forth. Just ask a tree about its purpose, and trust the answer you receive.

Trees can also perform physical healings. If you feel tired, ill, or injured, simply lean your back against a tree. You can choose whether to sit or stand. You'll immediately feel the tree begin to absorb toxins, pain, and low energies. It is a wonderful process! And don't worry—this won't hurt the tree. Just as they are able to transmute carbon dioxide into fresh oxygen, so too do they transmute and purify old pain energy.

Flower Therapy

Because we often forget to ask for help, Mother Nature has cleverly provided us with flowers to remind us. They are physical representations of love from our Creator and signs of the heavenly presence that surrounds us. When you work with flowers, it's like you're giving the angels a permission slip to intervene in your life. Until they receive this, they are unable to help you; they must stand on the sidelines and watch.

As you go through your day, you might suddenly notice a single blossom peeking out from a crack in the sidewalk or the magnificent blooms in a neighbor's garden. You might never have noticed them before, yet today they captivate you. The angels say that in these cases, the flowers were placed there just for you as part of their sacred purpose to heal you. As you pause and acknowledge the presence of the angels, you give them permission to help. So take a moment to literally stop and smell the roses. Your mind will become clearer and more focused, and you will be supported on your healing path.

At times you may become overwhelmed with the chaos and drama of your everyday life. These feelings appear as a psychic fog within your aura, making it very difficult to tell which way is up, what direction is forward, and where you want to travel. The sensation of pain is heightened, and all you can see is the worst in your situation. When you welcome flowers into your environment, negative energy is instantly lifted, alleviating your pain.

Beginning to work with flowers is as easy as bringing fresh blossoms into your home or planting seeds in your garden. Pictures are also just as potent as the fresh blooms. You can use images as a healing tool to surround yourself in positive, uplifting energy. We've been guided to use flower pictures as desktop backgrounds, phone backgrounds, and meditative art around our home. You can always take a moment to look at the image when you're in pain and call upon your angels. (For more in-depth ways to connect with the angels of nature, please see our book *Flower Therapy*.)

There are a few flowers that we recommend in particular for healing:

— The best is the **white rose**, which is connected to Archangels Michael, Raphael, and Metatron. It brings you clearing, healing, and balance across the board. When you bring a white rose into your home, it will uplift the energy, release all darkness and tension, and purify you. We love to use the white rose as a wand; wave it around your aura, especially over your areas of discomfort. You might feel it in your body as the pain is extracted. To allow yourself to surrender to the moment even more, have a loved one carry the rose around your body. (In Chapter 11, we share a more in-depth clearing ceremony that uses the white rose.)

You can also place a picture of the white rose in your pillowcase or under your mattress. As you sleep, the rose releases all pain from your body and aura. It will also work to clear negative emotions. By having an image of a white rose on your cell phone, you can easily clear yourself anywhere, anytime.

— **African violets** are wonderful to have in your living room, bedroom, or office. They purify the energy of the environment, making it more comfortable for your sensitive soul. If your surroundings are filled with toxins and heavy energy, you can experience more pain than usual. Have African violets around your home or workplace to ensure only positive energies can dwell there. Images of the violets work beautifully, too.

I (Robert) have grown to have such a deep appreciation for these little flowers. I keep them in my clinic and my home. I'm not yet an expert on growing them, but I've found that they are happiest when you keep them on a rotation of one week indoors, one week in a shaded area outdoors.

— **Calendula** helps clear pain by preventing the negative energy from ever reaching you. It serves as a preventive treatment and reduces the severity of pain, especially if it's coming from psychic attack. By drinking calendula tea, you strengthen your aura and create a shield of energy around you. Nothing negative can enter, but pain can still leave.

Lower vibrations can be transmitted through e-mails, over the phone, or through social media. Protect yourself from the negative energy that results by placing an image of calendula in your workplace or home office, or as your phone background.

— **Freesias** bring confidence and courage. They give you an emotional backbone but also strengthen your physical spine. Plant these flowers in your garden to affirm a strong, supported spine and painless body.

Singing-Bowl Healing

Singing bowls are instruments designed for healing and meditation. The sound is something like rubbing your finger around the rim of a wineglass, but on a larger scale. The most common are Tibetan bowls or crystal bowls; both are equally effective in creating sound vibrations that dissipate negative energy.

As we've discussed, negative energy is a home for pain to dwell. You can find a practitioner who works with the singing bowls or do so yourself. We suggest trying them out first; make sure they resonate with your energy and that you feel the benefits before investing in them.

When you hear the bowls, you instantly shift into a state of relaxation. Your breathing calms and your mind slows. You become a receptive vessel for healing energy. Playing the bowl for just a few minutes makes a profound difference. Afterward, you might like to close with a healing statement:

"Angels, please send me all the healing energy you can. I am willing to receive your guidance and energy, as I trust in your methods. I know you will take good care of me and guide me onto the path of wellness. Please help me feel good, relaxed, and completely comfortable within my body. Thank you."

Chakra Clearing

As mentioned in the previous chapter, your chakras are your centers of life force and vital energy. They are like sponges that absorb any type of energy, so they may contain things that are not for your highest good. To ensure that you hold only positive and loving energies, it is wise to clear your chakras. This is also an excellent way of purging your system of toxins. Chakras are like air conditioners in that they suction energy in while simultaneously sending it out. And like the filter on the air conditioner, your chakras can become dusty and clogged with negative vibrations. By clearing away this psychic debris, you'll ensure your chakras function in perfect balance.

Chakra clearing purifies your body of negative energy and the vibration of pain. It makes more room for comfort, peace, and tranquillity. Remember the image of your body as a closet that we mentioned in Chapter 3? If the shelves are filled with old, useless junk, there is no room to put exciting new items inside. The same is true for your body. Clear away the negative energy so you can replace it with vitality and well-being.

The following is a clearing method offered by Archangel Metatron, the biblical prophet Enoch who ascended into the archangel realm to become the guide of those newly upon the spiritual path. Archangel Metatron brings balance to all areas of your life. He helps correct disproportionate allocations of work, rest, and play, and maintains an energetic and spiritual balance within your chakra system. Whenever you feel stuck, blocked, or "clouded," call upon Archangel Metatron for healing.

Archangel Metatron's Sacred Beam of Light

Find a quiet space and begin by breathing deeply. Close your eyes and relax. Call upon Metatron by saying:

"Dear God and Archangel Metatron, please cleanse and balance all of my energies and chakras with your Sacred Beam of Light. Purify my body of pain, and replace it with comfort."

Visualize a beam of pure white light coming toward you from Heaven. Relax and watch as Metatron guides this healing energy in through the top of your head. See or feel yourself filled with light. Sense this energy filling all of your cells with the purity of angelic love. You may see ancient symbols being sent through the beam; if so, allow them to work their healing magic within your soul. You may recognize some of the figures, while others may be new to you. It's not important for you to understand everything. Instead, trust in the angels and God.

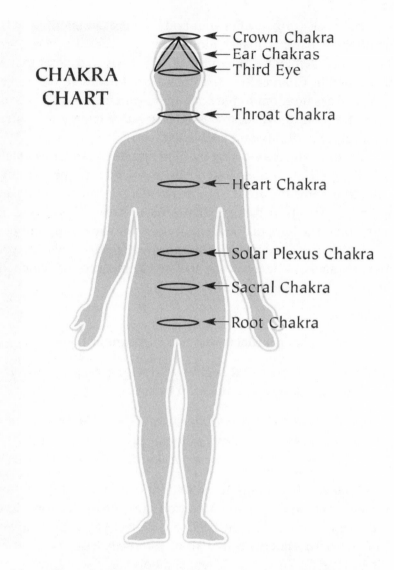

**CHAKRA
CHART**

← Crown Chakra
← Ear Chakras
← Third Eye

← Throat Chakra

← Heart Chakra

← Solar Plexus Chakra

← Sacral Chakra

← Root Chakra

Now, allow the beam to pass through your root chakra, at the base of your spine. Notice as it transforms into a ruby-red color. This light clears away blockages and fully awakens this chakra.

When the clearing is complete, Archangel Metatron will guide the beam through your sacral chakra. Here it takes on a vibrant orange. Feel the light dissolving all darkness and healing you.

Continue working with Metatron through the rest of your chakras:

- **Solar plexus**—yellow
- **Heart**—green and pink
- **Throat**—sky blue
- **Ear**—red-violet
- **Third eye**—dark blue
- **Crown**—purple and white

When you feel ready, thank Metatron by saying:

"Thank you, Archangel Metatron, for this healing and clearing.
Please continue working with me as I release all old energies that
have delayed my healing. I am now ready to embrace comfort
as the next chapter of my life."

The more you work with this method, the smoother and faster it will become. Initially, it may take five minutes or more for each chakra center. With regular clearing, there's not as much stagnation and psychic debris to remove, so you can move through the entire process in just a few minutes.

As the Law of Free Will dictates, the angels must have permission before they can assist you. Using this method allows Metatron to clear away negative energy whether you're aware of it or not.

෧ ෨

CHAPTER TEN

SPIRITUAL HEALING METHODS

Everyone has the ability to work with Heaven, and you don't
need special training or prayers to do so—the love in your heart is
all that's required. The angels say that everything that comes from
a place of love contains healing energy.

Healing may take many forms. It might start as a thought or
urge to make a needed change. Make a commitment to trust your
intuition, then ask for guidance from Heaven. Healing through
Divine aid can be instantaneous. Many have felt miracles occur
as they were praying for help, as you'll read about in this chapter.
Other times, people have been guided to the perfect therapy, practitioner, or natural solution to their problem.

When you surrender to the moment, the angels can do their
best work. Sometimes it's only when you give up the reins that a
situation can be resolved. When I (Robert) began healing with the
angels, I was accustomed to running my own therapeutic sessions.
So when the angels sometimes gave me clear directions to stay out
of the way, I was shocked. They told me that resistance, and having expectations of how the healing will flow, can actually slow
down the process. The best thing to do is to release control and
allow the angels to do their work.

In this chapter, we will explore the different ways in which we
can ask for Divine help to soothe our pain.

Calling On Your Angels

You, like everyone, have angels with you. They are a part of your physiology, as essential as any other part of your anatomy. Just like you're born with a heart and lungs, so too are you born with angels. Yours have been with you since *before* you were born, and they know you better than anyone else on this earthly plane. They were with you when you chose this life, and they know what purpose your soul carries. The angels are created from God's pure Divine intelligence and healing love. These beings of pure love and light surround you and guide you along a path of peace and fulfilment.

Angels are nondenominational, and help everyone equally. A very important point is that *the angels don't want to be prayed to or worshiped,* and they give all glory to God the Creator. You can call upon angels for aid because God created them to help us through our earthly existence. You can work with the angels in conjunction with Jesus, saints, or your personal religious preferences.

Your angels want nothing more than to help you. However, as we've mentioned, the Law of Free Will means that they cannot intervene in your life without your express permission. You must ask for their help. You don't need to know any special words or prayers—just thinking, *Help!* is enough. Make a commitment to call on your angels every day and allow them to assist you.

Of course you have the free will to completely ignore the Divine messages you receive. Nevertheless, we pray that you listen, and that more people begin to listen to their angels each day. As we all listen to the guidance from above, the world becomes a lighter place. You'll find opportunities for healing, achievement, and love when you tune in to the voices of the Divine.

༄

There are three different types of angels: *angels, guardian angels,* and *archangels.*

— There are an unlimited supply of **angels** that you can call upon. As you ask for healing, you're tapping into the boundless store of God's love to help you or someone else. The important thing to acknowledge is that you're never taking angels away from another person. These angels are continually streaming down from Heaven to be with us here on Earth. If you feel guided to send 100,000 angels to a person or environment, you're not reducing the supply of healing beings. Instead, you're surrounding that part of the world with such a bright light that its healing effects ripple out, defying the restrictions of time and space, and enhancing the lives of anyone willing to receive it.

— **Guardian angels** are your personal angels. They are a little different from deceased loved ones, who, while angelic in nature, can't technically be classed as angels. While you might hear people say that they feel that their grandmother is their guardian angel, the major difference is that angels have never been on Earth and have no ego.

Your guardian angels want you to succeed. They give you gentle pushes toward the path of least resistance. They remind you of your purpose and ensure you complete your soul mission in this lifetime. These angels were with you the moment you signed your contract for this life, so they know the true purpose for your time here on Earth. They may also help you learn the cause of your physical pain.

Your guardian angels know you better than anyone else and are the best friends you can ever have. Take time now to call upon them. Ask them to give you signs of their presence by saying:

"Dear God, thank You for sending guardian angels to me. Guardian angels, thank you for your constant love and support. I sincerely appreciate all that you do for me, even when I forget to acknowledge you. Please make yourselves known to me by giving me clear signs I will easily notice and understand. I would love to know your names, and I trust that as I hear names three or more times within this week, it's a sign from you. I love you."

— Our third group is the **archangels**, who are like the managers of the angelic realm. They are slightly larger and have more of a commanding presence than the others. For healing, we work with trustworthy and reliable Archangels Michael and Raphael. We also occasionally work with Archangel Metatron for certain types of healing.

- Archangel Michael, whose name means "He who is like God," is a very large and powerful archangel who is a protector. Archangel Michael heals by releasing the effects of fear and negativity from our minds, emotions, and bodies. Michael gives us courage, faith, and confidence.

- Archangel Raphael is a gentle yet powerful archangel who specializes in emotional and physical healing. Originally described in the non-canonical biblical Book of Tobit, Archangel Raphael is a saint in some Christian faiths. He has long been regarded as *the* angel of healing.

- Archangel Metatron is one of two human biblical prophets (the other being the prophet Elijah, who became Archangel Sandalphon) who ascended in a chariot of fire into the archangel realm. Metatron was the prophet Enoch, who lived such a pious, angelic human life that God transformed him into an archangel. Archangel Metatron guides those who are new to spiritual life, including spiritually gifted children.

Depending upon your religious beliefs, you may also want to call upon Jesus, Mother Mary, or healing saints, in addition to God and angels. We believe that the more heavenly intercession, the better.

The Supreme Healer: Archangel Raphael

Of all the archangels, Raphael (whose name means "God heals") in particular helps beautifully with relieving pain. He addresses physical, emotional, and spiritual concerns. When you call upon Raphael, you give him permission to bring healing to every area of your life, to every issue and blockage. His light can combat any negative thinking or perception of pain. By allowing him access to your body, you can remove suffering in all its forms.

Raphael heals with an emerald-green light of love. This energy has its own intelligence; it knows the areas that need the most help and naturally flows to where it's required. You don't need to do anything to assist it. Indeed, the best thing you can do is get out of the way and let the angels do their work. Surrender to the process and allow yourself to heal.

Call upon Archangel Raphael by saying:

"God and Archangel Raphael, please heal me. I ask you to release all forms of pain from my body and aura. I trust you, and I allow you to do your sacred healing work. Thank you."

ᕬ

Asking for Raphael's healing assistance can bring remarkable results, as Teresina Diaz learned. She already watched for personal messages from the angels in her everyday life. One of these signs was feathers. Teresina often found them around her car, on her balcony, and even inside her house! She knew that finding all these feathers in a short period of time meant that the angels were telling her to be prepared—she would soon be called to action. She chose to let go of fear and surrender to the situation. She knew that if she followed her guidance, everything would be okay.

In July 2013, a dear friend of Teresina's was diagnosed with breast cancer. A week after Teresina was given this devastating news, she found a large group of feathers on the pavement next to her car door. While she was used to finding one or two feathers, like a heads-up from the angels, seeing so many made her slip into panic mode. The large number of feathers was a Divine sign that something major was about to happen, but also reassurance that everything would be okay.

Initially, Teresina tried to dismiss her intuition. She told herself that perhaps a bird had simply met an unfortunate end. But the following week, she found feathers everywhere! There were feathers on her balcony, at the entrance to her apartment, near her car, and inside her home. She finally accepted that the angels were sending her a message, and thought it was a sign to tell her that her friend would be okay.

One day, Teresina noticed that her eye hurt whenever she looked at a light. That night, she couldn't sleep because of the pain. She canceled all her appointments with clients for the next few days because her eye was red and swollen and getting worse. A couple of days later, she was in agony. She didn't have health insurance but knew she had to go to the hospital. Her Earth Angel son, Erik, came to the rescue and drove her.

When Teresina and Erik arrived at the hospital, the doctors could tell the problem was serious. They wanted her to have emergency surgery, but something told her to wait. She heard a voice as clear as day whisper in her ear, "If you stay, then you will lose the eye." So Teresina decided to visit her parents in Mexico, and allow her eye to heal on its own. The doctors gave her antibiotics and sent her on her way. (In hindsight, she realized that not having health insurance made this decision easier. However, delaying emergency surgery is a decision that should not be made lightly or without support.)

Whenever Teresina returned to Mexico, she often smelled the fragrance of flowers, which is a common sign that your angels are nearby. During this trip, the scent was so strong that people would stop her to ask what perfume she was wearing! Teresina realized then that the feathers she'd been finding were signs for her, personally, rather than her friend. They were reminders to her that God was helping her and that all would be resolved.

In this peaceful environment, Teresina was guided to the perfect doctor, another Earth Angel, who also believed in the healing power of Heaven. This angelic doctor found that a previous operation to fix Teresina's nearsightedness had released an aggressive form of bacteria in her eye. Because the previous doctors had seen her when the infection was severe, their opinion had been that she needed an operation to prevent her from losing her sight. This new doctor suggested that she continue with the antibiotics she had been given, as well as positive thinking and energy work.

Teresina prayed that God and Archangel Raphael would help her and heal her eye. One night, she felt the archangel take her to an emerald temple. She was guided to lie on an emerald-green healing bed. The angels took a laserlike instrument made of clear quartz crystal, pointed it at her eye, and shone a golden ray of light through it. She felt Archangel Michael standing nearby and holding her hand.

Four weeks later, Teresina's eye was completely healed, with no more discomfort. Her doctor and family were thrilled with her speedy recovery. She regained her sight and now looks at life with a different perspective. She trusts in the healing power of the angels more than ever and spreads the word by teaching others.

ᘯ

Sometimes, healing miracles occur when people decide that pain no longer has a place in their lives. In July 2006, Andrea Kingsbury was diagnosed with Lyme disease, a serious illness that is transmitted through tick bites. It affected her both physically and neurologically, giving her pain and fatigue. At times she felt like she'd been run over by a bus, and she wanted to sleep all day. One side of her face became partially paralyzed! She was put on a series of antibiotic treatments, but the effects of the disease lasted for months.

There were times when Andrea felt well, but sooner or later she would fall ill again. It was devastating to her as she tried to raise her young children. Andrea finally got to the point where she couldn't take it anymore. It had been seven long months, and she refused to be sick any longer—it was time to become well.

A few weeks after this decision, Andrea was in one of her "feeling better" periods. She was in Florida on vacation, awake just before dawn, when a beam of emerald-green light suddenly struck her! This distinct color allowed Andrea to know that Archangel Raphael was answering her cries for help. The light surrounded her, and she could feel herself healing. Then, abruptly, it was gone. Andrea wondered if this amazing event would be repeated.

The next morning, just before dawn, the same thing happened. Andrea felt the emerald light healing every cell within her body. She heard a voice say what she had already felt: "You're healed."

To this day, Andrea has not had a single relapse of her Lyme disease, and rarely even gets sick! Before this experience, she used to have constant infections; now they are a thing of the past. Originally, Andrea was frightened of sharing this experience with others, but with the support of her angelic Reiki master, Carmen Carignan, she grew stronger and found the confidence to tell her story.

⁀

The angels can heal you only as much as you allow them. It's important to let go of your expectations, and be willing to let the best possible scenario unfold. Sabrina Muenzer from Austria healed her eye pain with the help of Archangel Raphael.

As a child, Sabrina was moved to the back row of her classroom, where she discovered that she could now clearly see the blackboard, which had appeared blurry to her from the front row. She raced home to tell her parents about this amazing improvement in her vision. However, instead of sharing her excitement, they took her to see an eye doctor, who diagnosed Sabrina with hyperopia, or farsightedness. Sabrina was not happy to be prescribed glasses! She resisted wearing them and took them off as often as she could.

Years later, when Sabrina was in her 20s, she suddenly felt a severe pain in her eyes and a headache while she was studying one night. She felt that all the reading she had to do at her university might have strained her eyes and caused this situation.

Sabrina chose to heal herself by working with Archangel Raphael. She committed to daily healing sessions where she called on her angels. She did this for five minutes a day, for about six weeks. Her pain steadily decreased until it disappeared completely.

Not only was the pain gone, but when Sabrina went to an eye doctor for a checkup, she discovered that she also no longer had any signs of farsightedness! Some people thought this was miraculous, but Sabrina knew it was simple for Raphael to do. Because she had not restricted herself to merely a release of pain, but instead allowed for a total healing, her angels were able to deliver it!

⁂

When Trey Handy granted Raphael full access to her body, it allowed for her healing to happen instantaneously.

Trey had been having problems with her right eye for a while; it was swollen, and it felt like pressure had built up behind it. Then one day, as she was looking out a window, her eye spontaneously began to water. She didn't know where this was coming from, but she chose to call on Archangel Raphael for help.

Trey sent out her plea while calmly standing in front of the large window. Immediately, she felt a strong presence behind her. She was frightened initially, but then she released her worries and said aloud, "Raphael, I trust you. I have no fear. Please do what you need to do."

Raphael had just been given the permission he needed. Trey remained still as she saw waves of light surrounding her. She was guided to sit down as she continued to see and feel energy surrounding her, rippling with white, purple, and flashes of green light. This wonderful experience lasted for several minutes, and Trey felt humbled.

Then she heard someone whisper in her ear, "This may hurt a little." She felt a pressure at the top of her head, like a rod being sent into her body and through her spine. A moment later, her vision was clear! Since that day Trey hasn't had any swelling, watering, or pain in her eye.

⟡

One day, Melodee Currier felt very ill. She had just read my (Doreen's) book *The Healing Miracles of Archangel Raphael,* so she decided to call upon God and the archangel for a healing. She held her head in her hands, closed her eyes, and visualized Raphael's signature emerald-green light. Her symptoms disappeared immediately, and when she opened her eyes, everything was that distinct green color. She instantly knew that Archangel Raphael was there and answering her prayers.

Since that moment, Melodee has had complete trust in Raphael, and he has always been there for her.

Archangel Michael's Spiritual Vacuuming

Vacuuming is a spiritual clearing method that is extremely effective for releasing fear and negative energy. Archangel Michael uses his etheric suction tube to remove blocks and counteract the effects of psychic attacks. At the other end of the tube is the Band of Mercy—a group of smaller angels who accompany Archangel Michael in his clearing work. They transmute all lower energies to a higher vibration and work to instill love and peace.

If your body is congested with lower energies, you can experience more physical pain. Invite Archangel Michael into your life and give him permission to help you. Ask him to vacuum your body, aura, or home, and he will remove unwanted negative energy for you.

People who have tried this method have reported dramatic changes. They say it as if a weight has been lifted from their bodies, and they have regained freedom of movement. They wake in the mornings with vitality and joy rather than fatigue. This high energy can inspire you, too, to create the changes you wish for yourself.

Archangel Michael can be with everyone simultaneously. You can call upon him for yourself, while also asking him to help loved ones. Remember, however, that Michael cannot interfere with others' free will, so he will only conduct healings if people are willing to receive them.

Call upon Michael for a spiritual vacuuming by saying:

"Dear God and Archangel Michael, please be here with me now. I ask you to please vacuum [me, my home, my office, my country, the planet, etc.]. *Please suction away the lower energy of fear. Release all darkness to reveal the light. Please release any pain from my body right now. I ask you to lift away all traces of negativity, leaving behind only love."*

In your mind's eye, see Michael clearing away the negative energy. By doing so, he reveals the beauty of your Divine light. He can also increase or reduce the intensity of the suction. Depending on your comfort levels, try asking him to switch the vacuum to low, medium, high, or extra-high. Continue working with Michael until you feel that all traces of fear are removed.

Then you can infuse the affected area with additional healing light. Say:

"Dear God and Archangel Michael, please send your loving, pure light of God into [my body, my home, my office, etc.]. *Please protect me from lower energies and remind me to call upon you for guidance and support. Thank you."*

When you undergo a spiritual vacuuming, you raise your energetic vibration. This makes it easier to understand the guidance of your angels. You may feel relief and also be guided to the right therapists. You may also find yourself aligning with more like-minded individuals.

⚭

The angels are happy to clear you as often as you need it, and they may also gently guide you to avoid situations that cause you pain. Vacuuming causes you to become a clean and clear vessel, which intensifies your sensitivity. Afterward, you may become more aware of which situations and people lower your vibration—when you're around them, you may notice headaches, fatigue, constant yawning, itchy skin, or difficulty concentrating. These are signs from your angels to extract yourself from these unhealthy situations or avoid the company of these individuals. For example, you may find that you can no longer listen to or be around people who complain a lot or who create lots of drama. By releasing those individuals, you're not being a bad friend—you're merely attempting to raise your own vibration. You're making the choice to allow only positive energies into your life.

As part of the natural process of developing your spirituality, you may also feel guided to modify other types of relationships. Your Higher Self may tell you to avoid alcohol and drugs, and the people who abuse them. Many people convince themselves that they're not addicted, but your inner knowingness tells you that their behavior is a form of self-harm. Trust this higher guidance. As a beautiful example of God's love, you have the ability to shine your light upon those in need, but you don't need to join others on their path of despair to do so. You can't help your friends if you involve yourself in their crises and dramas. Doing so will only create more people in need of healing.

Cutting Etheric Cords with Archangel Michael

Etheric cords are negative, fear-based attachments. From a clairvoyant standpoint, they look like tubes connecting you to other people, places, or objects. While they start out thin and string-like, they grow as time progresses and the relationship develops. They make you feel fatigued and are often responsible for unexplained pain. If there are no clear physical causes for your discomfort, it may be due to an etheric-cord attachment. Many people have experienced instantaneous relief after cutting these cords.

Etheric cords can both transmit and absorb low energy. Think of friends who are draining, or people who make you feel physically and mentally exhausted. This is due to fear-based cord attachments suctioning away your vitality and giving it to others. These individuals keep themselves going by siphoning off your energy reserves! On the other hand, another person's anger or stress energy can tumble down the cord *to* you instead. These emotions may hit you quite suddenly; one minute you're fine, and the next you feel intense anger or hurt. This can lead to sudden physical discomfort for no apparent reason.

Cords frequently attach to helpers. If you enjoy assisting others, or have a healing business of some sort, you may have etheric-cord attachments. That's why it's so important to cut your cords regularly. Otherwise, you may be overcome with negative attachments, which will drain you and make you feel chronically fatigued and burned-out.

The underlying energy of cords can stimulate thoughts and feelings such as:

- *What if they aren't there the next time I need help?*

- *I'm jealous. I want what they have.*

- *They made me feel so good. I need them in order to feel that way again.*

- *I don't want them to leave me.*

- *I resent them.*

- *They're the source of my power.*

- *They're the source of my healing.*

Archangel Michael can sever these cords of fear, releasing you from the unhealthy part of a relationship. To start this process, find a quiet space and begin by breathing deeply. Consider lighting a white candle for purification or sitting in front of a bouquet (or picture) of white roses.

Bring your attention to your physical body. Notice any areas that feel tighter or more restricted. Become aware of places that feel warmer than others.

Now take your dominant hand (the hand you naturally write with), and move it around your body to scan your aura. Pay attention to changes in air pressure, tingling, or heat. All of these sensations are clues that there are etheric-cord attachments.

Call upon Archangel Michael by saying:

"Dear God and Archangel Michael, please sever and release any cords of fear. I am willing to let go of this unhealthy, unbalanced energy. I choose instead to align myself with love and light. I ask you to remove negative energies from my body. Please release all attachments to pain. I am willing to heal. Please release all effects of these cords now. Thank you."

Follow Michael's energy throughout your body. Be aware of the areas of tension that are being dissolved.

You may receive intuitive flashes of the people or situations that those cords were connected to. Let these feelings move through your body, and release them. This is all part of the process. The angels recommend that you view the people you were attached to with love. It doesn't help to send them negative energy in return. Instead, dissolve the fear-based attachment and allow healing to transpire.

On occasion you may be randomly contacted by a person whose negative attachment you have cut. He or she may not be consciously aware of what happened, but you will feel the difference in your connection. You have let go of the unhealthy part that bound you, and all that remains is light, peaceful love energy. Remember, this process removes only the negative parts of these relationships—you can't ever cut the cords of love.

If you feel that certain cords were not released, ask your angels why. They may send you images or feelings about the person connected via this cord. Then, visualize a peaceful conversation with this individual. Say everything that's on your mind and in your heart. You may get a sense of what this person would say in return. Afterward, tune in to your body again. Notice the subtle differences and the greater energy you now feel. You've successfully released a negative, unbalanced relationship! Tell the universe that from this moment on, you will accept only loving people into your life.

The Power of Prayer

When you pray, you are connecting to the Divine consciousness that surrounds you. In truth, God is always within you, so you have the power to call on this potent energy no matter what. As we've said, due to the Universal Law of Free Will, the angels need to be granted access in order to intervene in your life. When you pray, you give them permission to step in.

Prayer doesn't require that you sit upright with your hands placed together and your head bowed. (Although if this is what feels right for you, then by all means, pray this way.) It's not a particular posture that gives prayer its power—nor is it the words! It's the underlying intention, the passion, and the heart that gives power to your prayers.

There have been a number of studies conducted on prayer that demonstrate its healing power. Some of these have been double--blind, which means that neither the physicians nor the patients knew which particpants were being prayed for and which were not. In most cases, the groups that were being prayed for healed faster, required fewer medications, and had a lower rate of complications after surgery.

We strongly rely upon prayer personally and professionally, and have seen its potent effects countless times. In our own surveys of people in pain, we found that those who healed the fastest were the individuals who called upon Divine intervention. They might have been desperate and grasping at straws, but they got on their knees and prayed for help. Finally, God and the angels had the "permission slip" they required. So if you're in need of healing, try prayer—it could bring you more relief than you can imagine. (For more information on the topic, we love and highly recommend books by Larry Dossey, M.D.)

There are two ways to pray: supplication (asking for something) and affirmation. There appears to be a slightly higher success rate with affirmative prayers. As an example, you might say in a prayer of supplication: "Please help me release this pain." In a prayer by affirmation, you would instead say: "My body is comfortable and fully healed." Notice the energy of those two phrases. Read them again and be aware of what each one feels like in your body. If you're sensitive, then you will likely feel a stronger resonance with the second statement.

Do your best to remove all negative and low-energy words from your prayers. Allow the change that you are praying for to ripple through every area of your life; don't pray, then complain all day about what you don't want! Do your best to clear those thoughts from your mind and silently repeat your healthy desire.

Some affirmative healing prayers to try are:

- "Thank you for my perfectly healthy body."
- "I am comfortable."
- "My body moves freely and effortlessly."
- "Regular movement is easy for me."

As you say these prayers, visualize God's healing energy and your angels surrounding you and giving you the support you need. There is no such thing as "praying too much." You can never irritate God or your angels; the sole purpose of their creation is to help you to complete your mission. They wish to fulfill their heavenly duties by guiding you to the healthiest way of being.

⟡

Kevin Hunter is an author who discovered the power of prayer on November 22, 2010, when he was put through his paces to learn about this immense healing energy. Although he had been spiritual his entire life, the following incident allowed his heart to fully embrace the Divine love surrounding him.

In early November, Kevin noticed that something didn't feel quite right in his groin. He was a little concerned, but not overly panicked, and began researching what it could be. His angels guided him to the answer that it was an infection, so he e-mailed his doctor to explain the situation and ask for antibiotics.

After several days passed with increasing testicular discomfort, Kevin went to the clinic. He explained that he knew there was a connection between his gym workouts and this growing pain, and again requested antibiotics. The doctor, however, said he would need to run tests first. As the doctor described the procedure, which involved sticking a tube into a place that it made Kevin very uncomfortable to imagine, he felt himself becoming nauseated.

The doctor suggested that it could also be Kevin's prostate, but then added that he was younger than the standard age when a person would begin regular checkups. This guess felt incorrect to Kevin, and he kept thinking about the angelic message he was receiving. He decided to skip the test, monitor himself at home, and return to the clinic if his symptoms didn't clear up naturally.

After a week, the pain had increased to the point where Kevin could barely move or walk. He could hear the voices of his angels loudly telling him what he needed, but he was fearful. *What if I have to go to the emergency room? What if they have to cut part of my body off?!* Kevin was panicked, overwhelmed by the many thoughts racing through his mind. His Higher Self told him it was merely an infection that could be cleared easily. His lower self imagined every outrageous scenario that would lead to devastating surgeries.

Kevin decided to e-mail his doctor, begging again for antibiotics. As a claircognizant (someone who receives Divine messages through thoughts and ideas), Kevin commonly got called a know-it-all, and he worried that maybe his doctor didn't like this direct approach. It probably felt unsettling for a professional to be instructed on what to do by someone with zero training. But soon, Kevin's pain was off the charts, so he called the doctor's assistant directly. The assistant said that the doctor had been traveling, and offered a referral to a urologist. The sound of that spun Kevin into a further panic. He hunted for another doctor to give a second opinion—anything to avoid the urologist! However, every practitioner he found was either booked or out of town.

Kevin's pain levels were starting to frighten him, but his lower self convinced him that if he went to the emergency room, it would be like a scene out of a horror film. So he finally gave in and requested an immediate appointment to see the urologist. Unfortunately, there were no openings for four days. Kevin's anxiety skyrocketed. *How am I going to make it? The pain is getting worse! It won't stop. Every day it climbs higher!* He spent his time waiting in bed, because every movement was followed by sharp, stabbing pain in delicate areas. When he walked, it was as if he faced the prospect of miles of hot coals and glass under his feet, with no hope for escape.

The day before Kevin's appointment, November 22, 2010, his life changed forever. It was the awakening moment that deepened his spirituality. On this day, Kevin drifted into meditation without effort and asked his angels for help. He was so used to doing everything by himself that asking anyone, even Heaven, for help was unheard of! He begged and pleaded with God and the angels. Having an honest conversation with them opened up every cell in his body. This was followed by the sudden, welcome release of his agonizing pain. Immense love took over his soul.

Kevin's clairvoyance opened up, and he saw his soul soaring through the bluest skies. He flew above heavenly white clouds where angels watched him. In the distance, he saw an extremely tall figure that looked like a stretched-out lamppost. As he approached it, his mouth opened in blissful awe. What he'd thought was a lamppost grew whiter and brighter, coalescing into a 30-foot-tall being with two gigantic, gorgeous wings! In a loud voice, the being said he was Archangel Michael, adding, "You will be fine. We're working on it." Kevin was filled with colossal joy and absolute trust in the archangel's words.

When Kevin awoke, his eyes were flooded with tears of joy, and he felt emotions that he had never experienced before. He felt his old life leaving him, and he was reborn with an entirely new outlook.

Kevin went to the urologist no longer full of fear of what would need to be done. He felt unusually calm about what might be ahead. The urologist didn't need to conduct any of the painful tests that Kevin had feared. He diagnosed Kevin with epididymitis, an infection in a tube in his testicle. He explained that it's common with sports players and athletic people. Kevin was shocked that this level of pain could be triggered by something as healthy as working out!

Kevin experienced an incredible improvement with every day that passed after the miraculous encounter with Archangel Michael. Although he had also received a ten-day prescription of antibiotics, he knew that it was truly Divine assistance that afforded him such a speedy recovery. By the second month, there were no signs of infection; it was as if it had never happened.

Kevin knew that something profound had taken place. This experience awakened him in ways he could never have imagined.

⊙∽

Trenia had experienced knee pain since her teenage years. Now it was preventing her as a mother from keeping up with her children. Although she'd tried physical therapy over the last 15 years, the pain never disappeared. She'd been poked and prodded more times than she could count. Prescription painkillers helped for only a short while before the pain eventually returned. The discomfort prevented her from exercising, which caused weight gain and further stress on her joints.

In early 2013, Trenia's knee worsened to the point where she couldn't put any weight on it. Any step she took resulted in her legs giving way. The doctors were convinced she had torn her meniscus, the essential cartilage within the joint. All of their tests confirmed it, and Trenia was scheduled to see an orthopedic surgeon for a meniscal repair.

This was a very difficult, emotional time for Trenia. However, in this moment, she remembered her angelic connection. She meditated and asked God and the angels to heal her knee. She didn't want to have the surgery, and she wanted to be there for her daughter's first theme park visit in a few weeks. She began receiving unmistakable signs and messages that this would be so.

Two weeks later, she underwent an MRI to confirm the location of the tear prior to surgery. However, the test revealed that there was no tear—her knee was completely healed! Her doctors said there was no longer any reason to do surgery. They had no explanation as to how her knee was able to heal the way it did, saying that meniscus tears do not have enough blood flow to repair themselves.

To this day, Trenia's pain is completely gone—and she had a great time taking her daughter to her first theme park!

❦

A beautiful soul named Sapphire healed her back through prayer. After a long day of cleaning her basement, carrying very heavy boxes and moving furniture around, she began to feel pain in her limbs and back. That night, the ache wouldn't allow her to rest, but she didn't want to take medication.

While lying in bed, Sapphire called upon Archangel Raphael. She asked for his help to release any pain and toxins from her body. In her mind, she saw two hands reaching down into her back. A warm and comforting golden light appeared, and Sapphire knew she was safe with these healing hands. Then, suddenly, she was completely pain-free! She was astounded by how quickly the healing came. Sapphire spent a moment thanking the angels for their help before peacefully drifting off to sleep.

❦

On June 3, 2012, Gina M. Adkins was moving into a new home in Arizona with her husband, Michael, and two young children, Alexis and Kaylee. Her mother and stepfather were there to help them move, too. It was a joyful day during what seemed to be a normal move. As Gina pulled a large, heavy box across the floor, she heard a *snap* and felt pain from her lower back shoot to her feet. After several hours of discomfort, she decided to lie down for a nap in the master bedroom.

An hour later Gina awoke to find herself paralyzed from the waist down. She screamed out for help, and her husband ran into the room. Gina had fallen from the bed to the floor. She cautiously rose to her feet on shaky legs, calling out, "Dear God, hear me now!" Michael carried her, arms and legs limp, into the living room, where the family looked on in shock.

Suddenly, a sense of peace rushed through Gina's body. She had a feeling that it would all be over soon. She looked up at her husband and said, "I'm fading." She felt a heavy weight lifting from her body as she drifted into an altered state. She heard her mother screaming, "Come back! Don't you leave us, Gina." In the darkness, she experienced an overwhelming sense of peace and joy. There was no pain, no worry, no heartache. She was realizing her Divine connection to God and the angels.

The next thing Gina remembered was opening her eyes to see a paramedic with piercing blue eyes—a blue she had never seen before in all her 35 years of life. He said, "My name is Hudson. You're going to be okay."

An ambulance rushed Gina to the emergency room at John C. Lincoln Hospital in Phoenix. Her heart rate was falling to 30 beats per minute—less than half of what it should be. At the hospital, Gina asked about Hudson, but no one knew about him. She became frustrated that she'd been sent back to Earth in pain, yet her rescuer was nowhere to be found. His eyes remained a vivid memory.

Gina needed to have a crash cart next to her for several days during her stay in the hospital. The cardiologist insisted she required a pacemaker to stabilize her heart. The orthopedic surgeon insisted that she have surgery to replace her ruptured L4 and L5 disks. Something within told her that those weren't the right options. Against all advice, Gina refused the surgeries. She continued to pray and ask God and the angels for healing.

Three days later she awoke at 2:45 A.M. to a whisper: "Stand now." She gently tried to sit up, and tears filled her eyes from the pain. Her feet touched the floor, but she wasn't sure that she could continue. Then she heard that voice again: "Get up for your children." She quickly stood up and walked to the hospital bathroom alone.

When Gina removed herself from the bed, alarms were set off, alerting the nursing staff. They rushed in and looked at her in amazement. They had thought she would never walk again! Eventually, Gina's heart began to regulate itself at 60 beats per minute. She continued making progress, walking more and growing stronger. Finally, she was able to go home a few days later. She thanked God and the angels for her second chance at life, but she couldn't stop wondering about Hudson.

Gina decided to write a thank-you card to the man who saved her life. She went to the fire station, card in hand, "To Hudson" printed on the envelope. The firefighter who answered the door remembered her. "You can walk?" he asked.

"Yes," she replied, "but I really need to see Hudson. He was with you that day you revived me."

The gentleman responded, "I am so sorry, but there was no man named Hudson with our crew that day. In my 11 years at the Daisy Mountain Fire Department, we have never had a Hudson working with us."

Gina thanked the firefighter and went back to her car. She looked up into the blue sky, tears flowing down her cheeks, and said, "I know You sent me an angel that fateful day. Thank You, God."

Now Gina is an avid walker and is preparing to participate in local 5K's for charity. Every day she walks two to four miles, feeling the presence of her angels by her side. She knows she is supported and is forever grateful for the healing she received.

႟

When all the following requirements are fulfilled, then healing will occur: give permission for the angels to help, listen for their guidance, take action steps, and express gratitude. If your loved ones give consent, you can pray for healing on their behalf, too.

Nicole would have stomach pain so severe that it occasionally led to vomiting. These bouts normally lasted one day, but sometimes they lasted longer. She compared the sensation to labor contractions! She would often be reduced to tears, as the pain wouldn't ease.

One episode had been going on for two or three days, with increasing intensity. Nicole lay in bed, losing hope; her healing methods weren't working. Her partner wanted to help, although he didn't have much spiritual knowledge apart from her occasionally talking to him about angels.

As Nicole lay there, she felt her body relax as she drifted off to sleep. While the pain didn't go away completely, she felt so much better. When she awoke, her partner asked if she felt different. She reported that she felt much better! He told her he had imagined filling her with pure white light. She was surprised by the gesture and impressed that he had come up with it intuitively. She thanked him and asked him to use it in the future if she was ever in pain.

Nowadays, when Nicole feels pain, she uses breath work and visualization. She inhales pure light and exhales stress, dark energy, pain, and anything else she want to release. She uses the prayer, "I breathe in Divine light, and I let go of pain. I am safe." Almost always the pain eases and is released from her body.

☙

Mariela Nikol no longer has any back pain thanks to the power of prayer. She attributes this to an invocation she found in a Bulgarian energy-healing book. She continues to repeat it every morning and evening with heartfelt emotion. Remember, the most important key with prayer is not the words but your intention behind those words.

A translated form of this prayer goes something like this:

"Dear God, Jesus, Mother Mary, and angels, please only see my per-
fection and not my mistakes. Please help me to awaken the natural,
self-healing quality of my body. I affirm perfect health in the name of
the light. Please do it easily and peacefully for the highest good of all."

Following the prayer, visualize your body being cleared from
the inside out. See a healing violet flame releasing all pain and
leaving behind only peace. Sense your angels surrounding you,
and the blessed Mother Mary encasing you in roses.

Mariela experienced almost instantaneous relief when she
said her prayer, and is pain-free to this day.

Miraculous Pain Prevention

Prayer can certainly ease pain, but it can also prevent it from
occurring in the first place. Rose Nickerson's miraculous story is
very touching—grab a tissue before reading it!

> I was in the hospital, very sick and afraid. I'd collapsed
> a few days before, and the doctors didn't know what was
> wrong. All the tests were inconclusive. My arms were bruised
> and swollen from all of the blood work and injections, since
> I'm petite, with tiny veins.
>
> It was early morning when a nurse came for another
> blood draw to see if I was bleeding internally. She was or-
> dered to take 15 vials! And because my arms were in such
> bad shape, she had to draw the blood from my hand—the
> most painful place to do it!
>
> I was afraid of needles and in so much pain that I cried.
> The nurse said, "I'm so sorry, but we have to do this." She
> gave me ten minutes to mentally prepare while she gathered
> her supplies.
>
> I'd brought the book *The Miracles of Archangel Michael*
> to the hospital with me and remembered reading that Mi-
> chael and Raphael work together. I said repeatedly, "Please,
> God and dearest Archangels Michael and Raphael, I ask for

your help in getting through this as quickly and painlessly as possible. Please be here with me now and negate my fear, anxiety, and pain!"

The nurse returned, told me to lie back, and raised my bed. I closed my eyes and envisioned Raphael's healing green light surrounding me. I felt Michael on my left side and Raphael on my right, holding my hands.

As the nurse drew the blood, I was astonished that I felt absolutely no pain. I was warm and calm, even serene, as she drew 15 large test tubes of blood from my hand. It took about 20 full minutes, and I didn't even twinge. I just lay back on my pillow and thanked God and the beautiful archangels for helping me.

Afterward, I told the nurse about my message to the archangels. She smiled at me and said, "They're always here for us. We just need to ask for their help."

Later that day, it was confirmed that I wasn't bleeding internally and that it was a bacterial infection that was making me so sick. I was treated and was able to go home two days later, with no more tests or needles.

Rose's story illustrates Archangel Raphael's remarkable ability to help those in dire need. He makes the seemingly impossible, possible. In desperate situations such as these, the only thing you can do is pray.

⁓

When Silvia's teeth became infected, her dentist recommended extraction. However, since her body couldn't tolerate anesthesia or sedatives, she had to call upon Raphael. She told her dentist to pull out her infected teeth without medication. He was against this decision, saying she'd experience terrible pain. But Silvia knew that it was the right choice, so the dentist finally agreed.

Two days before the extraction, Silvia focused upon meditation, prayers, and communing with God and Archangel Raphael. She asked him to protect her from pain and complications.

The day of her extraction, Silvia told her dentist, "It will be okay. I won't be here; I'll be in the woods." They both laughed, and as he prepared to extract her teeth, Silvia visualized green energy and light from Archangel Raphael.

After two yanks, the teeth came out—completely painlessly! The dentist was impressed, and told her that he didn't understand how it was possible. She explained a bit about meditation and encouraged him to try it. The wounds healed rapidly afterward.

Silvia says, "I know now how truly connected I am to Archangel Raphael."

Hands-on Spiritual Healing

There are many types of spiritual healing available. Each one has its own terms, qualifications, and methods; in truth, however, they are all one. The angels say it is like water coming from a showerhead. To us, they may appear to be individual streams of water, but in reality, they are all coming from one source. If the spiritual healing is anchored in the Light, it will be coming from our Creator.

During a spiritual healing session, practitioners channel Divine energy from the universe and into you. They shouldn't be using their own energy. Instead, therapists should step out of their egos and allow the healing energy to go to the areas in which it's needed most, according to God's infinite wisdom.

Spiritual healing isn't to be used to diagnose—only medical professionals can do this. However, it can be an excellent supportive tool for managing pain. Allow your intuition to guide you to the right practitioner. Only see healers who are happy and inspiring. If you feel drained or exhausted following a session, consider finding someone else.

Spiritual healing can include flower or crystal therapy, which we mentioned earlier. All the energies work together beautifully, and the treatment is tailor-made for you. Following their own guidance, healers may place their hands on the body or just above it. Physical contact isn't important, because they are working on an energetic level. You can even have spiritual healing performed over a long distance, as the energy of God is limitless. It can travel through time and space to be with each of us simultaneously.

A spiritual healing session is like a spa session for your soul. It recharges the batteries and activates your body's innate wisdom. It helps your mind to process the signal of pain and react appropriately. It connects you with your angels more easily, so that you can hear, feel, see, or just "know" their guidance. Whatever form it takes, you will be able to tell when a message is Heaven-sent. You may get information about your diet, career, relationships, fitness, finances, or another concern that may be linked to your pain.

☙

Spiritual healing can release even long-term pain in miraculous ways, as Saskia Gingrich discovered. Saskia was in three car accidents within the space of 18 months. The first two accidents gave her mild whiplash and a fractured wrist. But in the last accident, she tore muscles all around her neck, leading to excruciating pain. She had to wear a neck brace for six months to achieve some level of comfort.

Saskia went to physical therapy four days a week, receiving massage, ultrasound treatments, and water therapy. Unfortunately, nothing provided any relief. The physician wasn't sure what else he could do for her. She could barely move her neck and suffered daily headaches and neck pain.

One evening, she called a friend, looking for some distraction from her pain. Her friend said she was about to see a medium, and Saskia decided to tag along, too. Although she had never been to a medium, she did believe in angels and communication with deceased loved ones, and was curious about what would happen.

When they arrived, they were met by a cute English couple in their 70s, who invited them into their living room and made them both very comfortable. Four other clients joined them, too. The man indicated he was the medium and his wife was a nurse and psychic healer.

The man began doing psychometry (picking up on the energy of metallic items such as jewelry) on objects his guests gave him, and described what health problems he saw. Saskia thought that he'd have an easy time diagnosing her with her neck brace. She was surprised when he ignored her whiplash and instead described her difficulty breathing; he said he felt that she had to lean forward to catch a breath. Five years earlier, she'd had surgery for spontaneous pneumothorax (collapsed lung). She nearly died and had been in the hospital for a month. Prior to her surgery, the only way she could breathe was to lean forward.

The medium then described a man standing behind her. He was tall, with bushy black eyebrows—her father. The medium heard him say, "Strength, Saskia. You must have strength." Those were the exact words her dad would use to try to comfort her!

At the end of the session, Saskia and her friend were invited to stay for a cup of tea. While they were sitting there, the man's wife said to Saskia that she could hardly think, as she felt Saskia's pain. Saskia replied that she was in constant agony. The woman asked if she could perform a psychic healing, with assurances that she would not touch her and that she could do no harm. Saskia consented; she figured there was no harm in trying something different.

The woman sat in front of Saskia and began passing her hands over her body, from her head down to her shoulders and back up repeatedly. Slowly Saskia felt heat coming from her hands. It grew more and more intense. Suddenly, she felt the pain miraculously leave through the top of her head! Saskia wept with gratitude and relief as the healing took place.

Two days later, she had another physical-therapy session. The therapist was stunned that she had recovered full range of motion in her neck! Her doctors could find no remnants of the debilitating injury she had endured for six months.

A few weeks later, Saskia tried to find the healers to thank them for giving her back her life, but they had disappeared. These Earth Angels were sent to help her and then vanished. Now Saskia has embraced her own healing gifts and intuition, and enjoys living a pain-free life.

๑

The body absorbs healing energy and reacts to provide maximal comfort. Sometimes that means people fall asleep in order to heal.

Emily Southall's daughter was complaining of a painful earache one night. Emily offered her conventional children's painkillers, but her daughter would not take them. Perhaps on an intuitive level, the girl knew they would only mask the pain. Emily tried to contact their homeopath for advice, but she was unavailable.

Her young daughter was screaming in pain, and Emily felt helpless. She paced the room, thinking of how she could help. Then she remembered her Reiki training that she recently completed!

She walked over to her daughter and lay her head on her lap. Carefully Emily placed her hands over her daughter's ears and called on the angels as quickly as she could. Within a minute her daughter had fallen asleep. She later awoke with a huge smile on her face, all pain gone.

๑

All spiritual healing methods can bring relief for both people and animals alike. Lisa Aston is an Australian Animal Reiki Practitioner and Animal Communicator. She discovered Reiki's pain-relieving qualities when working with her animal companions.

One of Lisa's first clients was a ten-year-old Siberian husky, Tang, who was suffering from multiple health issues. He had lower motor neuron disease, epilepsy, pancreatitis, throat cancer, and a large mass in his stomach. As a puppy, Tang had been given a life expectancy of less than two years. Maria, his owner, had exhausted every veterinary, naturopathic, and herbal treatment available. At the time Lisa was contacted, a specialist had just given Tang three more weeks to live. To say that Maria was devastated would be an understatement. How could she continue without her dear friend? Although Maria knew that she should focus on mitigating her dog's pain, in her heart she hoped for a cure.

As Lisa entered Maria's home, her heart sank. The big husky could barely stand on his legs, and needed her assistance to lift his back end. His eyes were tired, and he was physically exhausted. Lisa was petrified; she wondered what she could possibly do to help him. (Later, Lisa would learn that "she" had little to do with the healing process. As she trusted in the Reiki and allowed the energy to flow, her clients would receive whatever they needed.)

Tang appeared to be aware of why Lisa was visiting. This was one of her most valuable lessons; her animal clients could intuitively know her true intentions. He lay quietly on the floor, in a space that allowed Lisa full access to him. She sat two feet away, then began her healing. She drew sacred symbols using her hands and placed them in his aura. He gazed at her with a look of gratitude and wisdom, a look that Lisa still recalls vividly.

Lisa was hesitant to offer hands-on healing because the dog's body was frail from dis-ease, though he bravely handled it without complaint. However, he kept looking at her and beckoning her to come closer. As Lisa inched forward, he kept his gaze on her until she placed her hands on the side of his body. For the next hour, Lisa intuitively moved around him, trusting where the energy was needed most. Tang relaxed into a deep sleep.

During her healing sessions with humans, Lisa would occasionally see visions of their lives. It gave her insight into her clients' health, and she would share these messages with them. This was the first time she has received these intuitive impressions when working on an animal. She resisted sharing what she saw at first, because she felt it might discredit her as a practitioner. Lisa saw fascinating visions of Tang in ancient China. His energy explained that in a prior life, he had been an emperor. Lisa called on her angels and chose to share these messages with Maria. It turned out that Maria had a deep passion for ancient Chinese history and had many books and videos on the subject.

Over the course of Lisa's sessions with Tang, he continued to share many more insights with her. He told her of things he loved to do, such as swimming in a particular place with crystal clear waters, eating ice cream out of a little bucket, and sitting in a child's wading pool. As Lisa shared all of this, Maria listened to and acknowledged his requests, taking Tang to the places she described. She laughed and said that Tang's ice-cream bucket was one of his favorite "naughty" foods.

Tang was ready to pass over, but he was waiting for Maria to accept it. Their love for each other shone through, and Tang's pain was eased by the treatments with Lisa. He became more comfortable as Maria began to heal, too. Tang passed away four months later.

Lisa still holds a special place in her heart for Tang and Maria. She knows that the healing sessions made a difference in their lives, and she learned in turn about the love that the animal kingdom has to share.

❧

Your own healing journey may inspire you to learn about many healing therapies. Keep in mind that spiritual healing can work wonderfully as an adjunct to conventional treatment methods, as Cindy Glavao learned.

Cindy had her first encounter with an angel when she was six years old, after she was hit by a pickup truck while crossing a highway in northern British Columbia, Canada. The impact threw her body across the highway into a ditch on the opposite side. Amazingly, she maintained consciousness after the accident, and when she looked up, she saw the most amazing sight. To this day, Cindy still remembers the magnificent colors of gold, pink, and purple. She saw sparkles of light of every color of the rainbow, and enormous auras that towered over here. Cindy sensed an incredible depth of love; in her heart, she knew that everything would be okay. She felt cared for in an indescribable way.

At the time Cindy didn't know anything about angels. When she later discovered the magical realm of angels, she learned that she was always Divinely protected in all ways. With the healing support of her angels, she experienced a comfortable and pain-free life.

Many years later, Cindy was devastated by the tragic passing of her young son. This led her on a spiritual journey to learn more about the angels, energy healing, and other topics. Eventually, she became a Reiki master.

During one of her healing sessions, Cindy had an incredible experience with Archangel Raphael. She was working on a young woman who was undergoing treatments for cancer. She'd come to Cindy for comfort and support while continuing with conventional treatments. Cindy was sending energy into the woman's back and visualizing her in perfect health when she suddenly saw the very same thing she witnessed all those years ago. She saw an intense green with sparkles of light all around, and clearly heard the words "This healing is done, and again it's done!"

Cindy knew immediately that this young woman had been healed. She felt an immense amount of gratitude and love, and had a hard time maintaining her composure. It was a truly moving and beautiful experience. That young woman is now in full remission. She lives a full and adventure-filled life as a firefighter while also going to school. Spiritual healing proved to be the perfect accompaniment to conventional treatments.

⚬⚬ ⚬⚬

CHAPTER ELEVEN

HONORING YOUR SENSITIVITY

Lightworkers are sensitive people who can be easily affected by others' emotional energy, even to the point of physical pain. A lightworker is someone who has a soul purpose to bring more light to the planet, whether through spreading joy, laughter, healing, or spiritual wisdom. There are many forms that a lightworker can take. For you, it may be as a parent to sensitive children, as a kind and compassionate friend, or as a healer and psychic.

Everyone comes to Earth with a soul-enriching life purpose. To bring about more enlightenment, you may have chosen to learn patience, how to deal with grief, or how to speak up in difficult situations. Some people, but not all, also come to Earth with a global purpose. These souls have chosen to have not just a personal purpose but also one that involves others. It may be advocating for animal welfare, bringing awareness of our food quality, or teaching spiritual workshops and introducing people to angels. These global purposes are gifts to sensitive souls who will follow the light to complete their important mission. Your guardian angels know what your purposes are. They were standing right by you as you signed the contract for this life. You chose the family to be born to, the experiences to have, and the lessons to learn. Under the watchful eyes of your angels, you can complete everything on that list.

Our egos are afraid of us fulfilling our purpose, because the ego is driven by fear alone. Your life purpose is to shine light and love through your career and other activities, and the ego knows that your purpose will eradicate fear. So your ego continually urges you to delay working on your life purpose. The ego distracts you with other projects, including physical illness or pain, so that you won't do all of the fear-lifting work that you are destined to do.

In fact, I (Doreen) found in my counseling practice that the bigger someone's life purpose was, the bigger the amount of fear he or she had! To put it another way, the more people you signed up to help, the louder your ego is going to scream, "No, you're not qualified! You can't help anyone! You're not ready! What if you fail?" and other untruths. The truth is that you *are* ready to help others, and you can do so even when your body doesn't seem to be 100 percent ready. In fact, all of your experiences with pain have made you extremely compassionate to others in similar situations. This makes you extra-qualified to help those who are suffering, because you know what it's like!

It may seem radical to think that we've chosen these situations for ourselves, yet we do so for the sake of growth. If we continue to do the same things we've always done, then we'll get the same results we've always gotten. Instead, we wish to challenge ourselves so that we can learn more, feel new emotions, and expand our souls' knowledge. It helps us to appreciate the contrast. As they say, only when it rains do we remember to be grateful for the sunshine.

If you resonate with this concept, you may be highly sensitive to energies. Pay close attention to your feelings in various situations. You may find that spending time with complaining, gossipy friends literally gives you a headache. This is because you're taking on the harsh energies of their words. Notice what days your pain is particularly bad, and notice whom you've been around. Notice what the energy felt like and the topics of conversation you took part in. These are all keys to understanding how to eliminate pain from your life.

Listen to your heart—it holds all the answers. When you ask your heart serious questions, it always answers with love. Ask it if certain people are enriching your life or if they are sending you negativity. The angels say that the people you spend your time with affect you in either a positive or negative way. Their energy interacts with yours and can create an uplifting effect, or a depressing one.

If you feel tired after being around certain people, avoid them. Keep your circle of friends filled with high-energy, happy people. Yes, we are human and are allowed moments of sadness. Yet when our hearts are filled with joy, we bounce right back up and focus on the light. So be courageous and release negative and draining people from your life. Perhaps try it for just a week; you'll notice the profound and healing difference that it makes. This may persuade you to try letting them go for a month, and then longer.

We don't blame these people for their harsh energy. Instead, we find that it becomes a moment to pray. We can focus our light upon them in the hopes that they will join us in a happy, high-energy, peaceful place. Imagine yourself much like a helium balloon—if you attach yourself to heaviness, it will always be hard to fly. If you choose instead to surround yourself with lightness, the possibilities become endless.

Psychic Attacks

Psychic attack is lower energy that's directed your way. It isn't as mysterious or dark as it might sound. There are no voodoo dolls, midnight rituals, or animal offerings. Psychic attack can be as simple as someone being jealous of you. It's often an unconscious thing. People aren't intentionally sending you negative energy; it just happens as they slip into their egos and have lower-energy thoughts concerning you. For example, perhaps you once purchased a new bag. As you went out to lunch with your friends, one of them wished she had your bag instead of hers. In this instance, she slipped into the energy of jealousy and inadvertently launched a psychic attack.

The physical sensation of psychic-attack energy is painful. Imagine knives, spears, bullets, axes, and other weapons that are created out of fear. The pain is very physical, yet the source is purely energetic.

This energy can lodge itself anywhere in your body. The most common places are around the shoulders. If you've had painful, tense shoulders for no apparent reason, now you know why! The lesson, however, is not to return the favor and send an attack back to the initial perpetrator. This would only continue the cycle of fear energy, which isn't something you want to exchange. Instead, send such people love. They sent you negative energy because they slipped into fear mode. If you surround them with loving thoughts and angels, they will become uplifted.

When we raise our vibration, we celebrate each other's success instead of trying to compete. In spiritual truth, there's more than enough for everyone. The angels show us images in which we are all born with a treasure chest, containing the same opportunities as everyone else on Earth.

It's up to you to decide whether you will open the treasure chest of your dreams or leave it sealed. Once you choose to open it, you will realize that there's no such thing as "luck." You deserve everything that comes your way. The more open and receiving you are, the more the angels can bring you.

Competing is a trap of the ego. It wants us to think that in order for us to have something, we need to take it from someone else.

Don't listen to this limiting voice; it will only bring you more pain. You have free will. If you no longer want the low energy of psychic attack to be connected to you, it can be released. Calling on your angels creates a high-energy clearing.

Unfortunately, it appears that the more successful, happy, and healthy you become, the more people seem to send psychic attacks. This is why it's so incredibly important to only spend time with loving individuals. These people will be proud of you and supportive of your journey. They will understand that just because you have something, it doesn't mean that they can't have it, too.

Psychic-Attack Clearing

Find a quiet space where you won't be disturbed. You can lie down, but we have found that sitting upright works the best. Sit on the edge of a bed or scoot forward on a chair. This way, your back and shoulders are free and easily accessible. Close your eyes and focus on your breathing. Take slow, deep breaths in and out. Continue this for two or three minutes to relax. There's no need to rush healing. Now call upon Archangel Raphael by saying:

"Dear God and Archangel Raphael, please be here by my side. I ask for your heavenly assistance right now. Please clear away any forms of psychic attack or lower energy lodged within my body and aura. I am willing to let this go and send loving angels in exchange. Help me to feel pain-free, relaxed, and supported. I know you will defuse all psychic attacks right now, painlessly and effortlessly. Thank you."

You may get sensations running through your body as Raphael conducts his healing. Just surrender to the moment, and allow your angels to do what they do best. You may get visions of the archangel pulling out the weapons of fear. Remember not to send this low energy to someone else. Allow the angels to clear it and transmute it to the high vibration of love.

If you get thoughts or visions of other people who may have sent you this energy, take a moment to send them some love. They are in need of it right now to uplift them to the higher energy of peace. Visualize a pink beam of light being transmitted to these people and dissolving all unhealthy aspects of your relationship.

Next visualize Archangel Raphael rubbing a soothing emerald-green gel in the areas where the psychic attack was removed. This balm instantly heals the locations on your body that felt pain. It also prevents the attack from returning for some time.

White-Rose Clearing

Purchase a fresh white rose from your local florist, or clip one from your own garden for an even stronger connection to the flower. The white rose is associated with Archangel Michael, who helps release negative energies; Archangel Metatron, who brings us balance and clears our chakra system; and Archangel Raphael, our supreme healer. So this one blossom is connected with three powerful archangels who all have a unified goal of helping and clearing you. By working with the white rose, you're inviting these angels to your side and giving them permission to heal you.

Find a safe space to clear this heavy energy from your aura. Once you're comfortable and prepared, you can begin. Say:

"I ask that this white rose please clear me of all lower energy.
I am willing to let go of any psychic attacks originating from others.
By doing so, I affirm peace for all involved."

Move the white rose through your aura, spending extra time over your head and shoulders, as this is where psychic-attack energy will commonly sit. As you wave the white rose around your body, you may feel various sensations, signaling that the negativity is released. (You can also have a friend or loved one move the rose about you.)

When you feel that the process is complete, you have two options. You can place the rose in a small vase or glass of water and allow it to continue clearing your room. Or you can ceremoniously toss the rose into the garden, giving the energy back to Mother Earth.

Crystals for Clearing Psychic Attacks

You can move specific crystals through your aura to eliminate lower energies and create harmony. As you purge negative vibrations, you release the pain that came along with them.

— **Selenite** wands are wonderful for clearing psychic attacks and can be purchased inexpensively. It doesn't matter whether the crystal is polished or rough—the energy is the same. As you slowly draw the selenite through your aura, you'll be pulling out all projections of fear. This is a great practice after spending time with negative people, or when you have been in a group setting. Selenite brings you strength, heals your insecurities, and shows you that you're Divinely powerful in all ways.

— **Amethyst** is an excellent psychic protector. You can move the crystal through your aura to release psychic-attack energy. It has the added bonus of transmuting low energy into the high energy of joy. All the things that no longer serve you can willingly be released in exchange for happiness. Let go of the old so there is enough room to welcome in the new.

Call upon your angels and place an amethyst crystal on your brow. This will eliminate those negative thoughts from clouding your future. The benefit of carrying or wearing amethyst is a continuous flow of positive thoughts that will shape your bright and positive future.

❧

Clearing the energy of psychic attack is something you must regularly do. We don't want you to become focused on negativity, but do check in with yourself frequently.

Shielding

Once you remove the energy of pain, you'll want to keep it away, so spend time strengthening your aura and shielding it. It would be a perfect world if we didn't have the need for shielding. However, not everyone has the same loving outlook on life that you have. Therefore, it's best to engage in this practice, especially before going to crowded places or events.

Some people think that shielding is a way of anticipating attack. They feel that it's an affirmation to the universe to send negative energy toward you. When we asked the angels, they said that it was just like locking your front door. If you leave your door open, it allows anyone and anything to enter. In closing that passage, you still have access to the little peephole on the door. You get to decide which vibrations can enter and which ones stay outside.

Your particular situation will determine how often you need to invoke your shield. A general guideline is to practice this twice daily: once in the morning when you get up, then again in the evening as you go to bed. Most shields last for approximately 12 hours. However, when exposed to harsh energy, your shield may weaken faster than normal. When surrounded by negative people or difficult situations, invoke your shield every hour, if needed. Ask the angels to give you clear signs that you need to shield yourself again. They may send you physical sensations, or the thought of shielding may just pop into your mind. Take a moment to do so, and notice the difference it makes in your day.

The following are all wonderful methods for invoking a shield.

Calendula Tea for Aura Protection

Calendula is wonderful at shielding and protecting your aura. It is a bright orange flower used in herbal medicine for healing wounds and clearing infection. When taken as a tea, however, its energetic properties shine through.

Drink a cup or two and you will feel stronger, more stable, and less influenced by others' emotions. It's an excellent travel companion in a to-go mug when visiting gossipy friends or group environments. You can be constantly shielding yourself, and no one will know what you are doing. Drinking a simple cup of tea is all you need to do to keep your energy pure and clean.

Angel Cocoon

Visualize a stream of miniature angels gliding down from Heaven. As they get closer, they begin to spiral around you. They start at the top of your head and float around your body—both front and back. They continue all the way down to the base of your feet, forming a never-ending connection from you to Heaven.

As the angels come close to you, they pick up and release negativity. Each one who leaves to take away this low energy is simply replaced by a new angel.

The angel cocoon is very cleansing and comforting. Often you'll hear giggling and laughter in addition to the sound of fluttering wings.

Amethyst Cave

Imagine that you're sitting inside a giant cave made of beautiful amethyst. You're surrounded by the protective purple light that the crystals emit. Every crystal point is absorbing lower energies from your body and aura, and detoxing you from heaviness and pain. Once all darkness is removed, the crystal points infuse your body with healing.

The amethyst cave awakens your intuitive abilities and strengthens your connection to the angels. This is an excellent meditation to do prior to visiting metaphysical fairs or giving speeches of a spiritual nature.

Rubber-Ball Shield

Archangel Michael stands over you, holding a bowl of liquid rubber that's cooling down. This is a special protective substance that deflects negativity and psychic-attack energy, causing them to bounce off like a ball. This shield is the same color as Michael's aura, royal blue.

Ask Michael to shield you by saying:

"Dear God and Archangel Michael, please encase me in a protective shield of rubber. Infuse this rubber ball with your sacred light. May any negativity bounce off, and all love be absorbed. Thank you."

Visualize Archangel Michael carefully pouring the royal-blue rubber over your aura. It will instantly envelop you in its protective warmth.

Mirror-Ball Shield

See yourself standing inside a mirrored disco ball. This shield reflects any negativity or destructive thoughts that may be sent your way.

It's perfect when you have meetings with others who may not have the best intentions.

Lead Shield

This shield invokes the strength of thick, impenetrable lead, infusing it into your aura. The lead is lightweight, however, so it's easy to carry around. Visualize metal permeating your auric field, which will give you an extremely strong defense.

This shield is best used when you feel frightened or unsafe. Invoke it as you walk home from work or catch late-night public transportation. People will sense your strength and leave you alone.

Color Shields

Each color has its own vibration, and you can intuitively choose one to blanket your aura with. Close your eyes—the first color that comes to your mind is the right one for this moment. Tomorrow you may be guided to the same one or a different pick. Trust this inner sense of knowing, and visualize your aura glowing with that color.

Here are a few of our favorite colors to shield with:

- **White** is a strong, pure energy of protection and clearing.
- **Purple** is excellent for psychic protection.
- **Pink** helps you protect yourself and comes from a place of love.
- **Gold** is a healing, as well as protective, energy.
- **Green** works well for a healing shield.
- **Yellow** is great for study and concentration.

❧

Your thoughts are shaping your journey ahead. Remember that you are creating your reality. Every thought is an affirmation for what you manifest. So if the path ahead of you seems frightening, painful, or disappointing, check in and see what influences have been flooding your mind. On the other hand, if it looks beautiful and perfect, you're doing a wonderful job maintaining high-energy thoughts.

Keep in mind the future you want to manifest for yourself. Choose your thoughts wisely, be careful with the company you keep, be diligent with your shielding, and clear your energy regularly.

❧ ❧

AFTERWORD

You were not put on Earth to suffer. You are here so that you can create greatness. If you forget about this, then you'll lose sight of the bigger picture in play. You're here because underneath the illusion of pain, you are inspiring. Already you create joy in the lives of others. Many rely on you for your open and warm heart. You might fail to remember this from time to time, but please recognize that you're more than a suffering body. Your soul is so powerful, and it's the very thing that's going to help you get through this next stage.

Sometimes pain has played a role in a person's life for so long, it is difficult to remember how to function without it. While this sounds bizarre, it's true for many. So think: What has pain prevented you from enjoying? When it is gone, how will you take back those opportunities and enjoy yourself each and every day? The goal here is to release the hold that pain once had on you. When you let go of this old companion, there is space for the heavenly energies of your angels. These beings of love shine the light on your path ahead. Your comfortable, safe, rewarding path. The path you were meant to walk.

The angels say to only go forward with the path of change if it aligns you with greater peace. If you make choices in order to "keep up with the Joneses" or because you feel unlovable, you are listening to the lower-energy voice of the ego. The ego wants to see you suffer and fail.

Please be mindful of which voice you're listening to right now. Are you uplifted, motivated, and inspired by your inner voice? Or are you shamed and blamed by the voice? The first is the voice of your angels; the second is the lower energy of the ego. You must constantly tune in to check which guidance you're listening to. Only one of them wants you to feel happy, healthy, and loved—make sure that you're aligned with *that* voice!

Make it part of your daily routine to invite your angels into your life. Give them permission to help you by saying something like the following:

"Angels, I welcome you into my life today. Please walk with me each step I take and guide me along my path. Please help me in any way you can. I am willing to receive all the guidance and healing you have for me. Thank you."

When you do this, your physical body will not only feel wonderful, but amazing opportunities will fall into your lap. Promotions at work, new friends, satisfying relationships, or other types of abundance may be brought onto your path. This is a natural process that comes with aligning with your Higher Self. You become one with the universe and are able to shine your light and express your gifts from God.

Know that all things about you are created perfectly. There are no mistakes made. How your body is and feels right now is all part of a greater plan. If there's anything you would like to be different, then now is your opportunity to change it—with help from God and the angels!

෧෨ ෨෩

APPENDIX

Specific Areas of Pain and Their Healing Methods

Here is a list of common areas of pain and their healing methods, including herbs, supplements, crystals, prayers, spiritual and energetic healing techniques, and other modalities. We also discuss possible energetic causes for the pain in these areas.

For best results, follow your guidance when assessing the methods and approaches below. Do not use all the therapies listed at once. It's best to try only one or two at a time so you know which ones are working. If you try five things simultaneously, you'll never know which healing method is doing the job.

If you're drawn to affirmations, aim to repeat them several times a day. Some people find it useful to set an alarm on their phone to remind them to take a minute or two to repeat their affirmations. The more you affirm your positive desire, the more your body believes it.

Allover Pain

Energetic Cause

You need to release the pressure. Right now your body is like a bottle of soda that's been shaken up. The pressure has built up inside and needs to be let out. As you open the lid, things may bubble up and get messy. But, almost instantly afterward, you become calm. Now is the time for you to let go and move closer to the peace you crave.

Natural Prescriptions

- Consider detoxing; your body may be storing harmful compounds.

- Take 25 drops of ginger tincture or 1,000 mg of ginger supplement, three times per day, to relieve pain.

- Take 1,200 mcg of SAMe daily—400 mcg three times a day—for two weeks. This is enough to pull you out of your slump and alleviate pain. Then you will have new perspectives and a positive outlook for the future.

- Take 4,000 mg of boswellia in two or three doses throughout the day. It will lift your spirits and clear any obstacles to your healing.

- Consume turmeric in food, and consider taking it in supplement form or as a tincture. It reduces inflammation and detoxes your body.

- Take 400 mg of magnesium per day to help relax general muscle tension and promote comfort.

- Have a vitamin D screening to ensure you aren't deficient. People with low levels tend to need higher amounts of pain medication.

- Take 10 drops of cramp bark three times a day to let go of tension.

- Take 2 teaspoons of corydalis for acute pain. The following day, take ½ teaspoon, in three doses throughout the day.

Spiritual and Energetic Solutions

- Clear your chakras with Archangel Metatron's Sacred Beam of Light. Make this part of your daily practice.

- Let go by performing a full-moon release ceremony.

Prayer

"Dear God and angels, please send me your healing light. Help me to let go of all issues from the past and embrace my health and wellness. I exchange pain and discomfort for love, peace, and joy. Angels, please open my heart so that I may heal. All that comes from love attracts the essence of healing. I call upon the healing angel Raphael to be with me now. Please bless me with your emerald-green light and heal every single cell. Please illuminate the light within my body so that only love can reside within it. Thank you."

Affirmations

- "I willingly release all pressure from my life."

- "Each step I take brings me closer to peace."

- "My body is my temple, and I treat it well."

Ankle/Foot

Energetic Cause

You're frightened to take the next step. The next part of your journey feels important, and you don't want to make a mistake. Don't allow that fear to delay your progress.

Natural Prescriptions

- Take 2.5 ml of devil's claw extract twice a day in a little water. It will nourish the tiny bones in your ankle and foot.

- Boswellia may be helpful to ease pain and discomfort.

- Consider acupuncture treatments.

Spiritual and Energetic Solutions

- Clear your chakras with Archangel Metatron's Sacred Beam of Light. This releases fear and gives you courage to move forward.

- Perform a white-rose clearing to remove any blocks to progress.

- Place an African violet in your office to cleanse the energy.

Prayer

"Dear God and Archangel Michael, please clear me of all fear energy now. I ask that I be filled with courage to take the next step. I know

that this moment is occurring because I am truly ready for it. I welcome this positive change into my life, and I release all that held me back. I willingly let go of all pain and discomfort and choose to fulfill my Divine destiny! Thank you."

Affirmations

- "It is safe for me to take the next step."

- "I am ready for what is to come."

- "I accept my purpose and choose to move forward now."

Arm

Energetic Cause

A fear of success. This could be your time to shine; please don't resist it!

Natural Prescriptions

- Take 2.5 ml of devil's claw extract twice a day in a little water. This will soothe the arm pain.

- Take 4 drops of Saint-John's-wort extract to heal the nerves in your arm.

- Take a relaxing sea-salt bath to cleanse your body of toxins.

Spiritual and Energetic Solutions

- Consider doing a full-moon release ceremony to let go of anything causing you pain. By releasing it, you allow the next chapter of your life to begin.

- Clear your chakras with Archangel Metatron's Sacred Beam of Light so you are willing to accept all the good in your life.

Prayer

"Dear God and angels, please take away all pain as I become comfortable with success. I trust in your process and know that now is the right time for me to shine. I relinquish fear and embrace the beauty ahead. Please show me how to achieve the next step in my journey. I allow you to lead the way. Thank you."

Affirmations

- "I am ready to fulfill my purpose."
- "Success greets me as I welcome it."
- "I allow my light to shine."

Back, Lower

Energetic Cause

Fears and worries about money. Difficulty moving forward after a traumatic experience.

Natural Prescriptions

- Take 4,000 mg of boswellia in two or three doses throughout the day. This reduces inflammation and clears blocks to healing.

- Add turmeric to the foods you prepare. You may also feel guided to take a turmeric supplement.

- Consider taking willow bark as an extract or tablet. This takes away inflammation and pain. It works well if the area feels hot or if the pain brings a burning sensation.

- Take 400 mg of magnesium each day. Magnesium relaxes your muscles and makes you feel like you've had a massage.

- Take 2 teaspoons of corydalis for acute pain. The following day, take ½ teaspoon, in three doses throughout the day.

- Take 10 drops of cramp bark three times per day to help you let go of pain and tension.

- Heal and balance the lower back with Bowen therapy or massage.

Spiritual and Energetic Solutions

- Place a garnet crystal in your pocket to carry with you during the day. This heals any imbalances in your root chakra and gives you a feeling of stability.

- Bring yellow lilies into your home to heal financial issues. They work to attract the energy of abundance.

- Call on Archangel Michael to cut etheric cords from your lower back. These energy attachments may be draining you. They may also be responsible for your discomfort and unexplained pain.

Prayer

"Dear God and angels, please clear away any and all pain from my lower back. I am willing to release this now in exchange for comfort. I allow the universe to provide for all my earthly needs, giving me security. I know I will always be safe under the watchful eye of the angels. I call upon Archangel Michael to erase all fears and concerns connected to money, safety, and security—now! Thank you."

Affirmations

- "My financial needs are always met."
- "I am fully supported as I move forward."
- "I confidently follow the direction of my guidance."
- "I willingly release the past."

Back, Upper

Energetic Cause

You may be the target of jealousy. Be mindful of the people you spend time with. There may be psychic-attack energy in your upper back. Anxiety about speaking up and saying the truth may be present.

Natural Prescriptions

- Relieve pain and inflammation with willow bark supplements.

- Take 400 mg of magnesium to help lift the weight of the world from your shoulders.

- Mix 1 teaspoon of turmeric powder with a small amount of yogurt or other food with fat in it. Eat this daily to reduce pain and discomfort.

- Take 2 teaspoons of corydalis for acute pain. The following day, take ½ teaspoon, in three doses throughout the day.

- Soften tension with Bowen therapy, massage, and acupuncture to allow healing to take place.

Spiritual and Energetic Solutions

- Work with Archangel Michael and practice regular spiritual vacuuming. It's likely you've absorbed negativity from others.

- Shield yourself daily to prevent lower vibrations from harming you. You may find shielding with purple and pink light to be highly effective.

- Carry an amethyst crystal with you to absorb and transmute all lower energies.

- Perform a white-rose clearing, concentrating on the areas around your shoulders and upper back. The white rose pulls out negative energy and pain.

Prayer

"Dear God and Archangel Michael, please shield and protect me from negative energies. I ask you to be with me and ensure my safety. Please give me the confidence to shine my light brightly without delay. Purify my body and lift out all forms of pain. Archangel Raphael, please fill my body with your healing. Thank you."

Affirmations

- "I am safe and Divinely protected."
- "Everything coming toward me is positive and good."
- "I confidently speak the truth."

Chest

Energetic Cause

A fear of revealing the true you. Sometimes you hide behind a mask and pretend to be someone you're not—at work, with friends, or even with loved ones. You are more lovable than you realize, and the world deserves to see your beauty.

Natural Prescriptions

- Take 800 mcg of SAMe in divided doses—400 mcg two times a day. This uplifts the soul and brings laughter and happiness.
- Take 400 mg of elemental magnesium each day to open your chest and heal pain.

- Try rubbing a drop or two of peppermint oil on your chest. It may cause some redness, but it should release pain and tight muscles quickly.

Spiritual and Energetic Solutions

- Call upon Archangel Raphael and ask him to heal your heart. The chest is the location of the heart chakra—the place you store old emotions and heartache. Raphael will cleanse this away with your permission. Say: *"Archangel Raphael, please help me heal my heart. Please release tension from my chest by clearing away old emotions. Thank you."*

- Ask Archangel Michael to take away the mask you have been hiding behind and reveal the true you. Say: *"Archangel Michael, please give me the courage to be the real me. I ask you to peel away the false layers I put in place to survive. Take off the mask now and let my true self shine through. Thank you."*

Prayer

"I know I can be but one person this lifetime—me! Dear God and angels, please help me to reveal who I am inside, my true self. Please give me the strength to break through this shell and become who I was born to be. I'm ready now. I let go of fear and all forms of pain as I embrace my inner truth. Thank you."

Affirmations

- "It is safe for me to be me."
- "Others benefit when I show my true self."
- "I reveal who I am inside."

Head

Energetic Cause

You analyze everything down to the finest detail. Sometimes this prevents you from making progress, as you need things to be absolutely perfect first. You strive for perfection and may get lost in details rather than experiences.

Natural Prescriptions

- Take 800 mcg of SAMe in divided doses—400 mcg two times a day. After a week or two, you'll find the cloud lifts from your mind. You will become happier and lighter as you release the shackles of pain.
- Willow bark tablets can serve as a handy headache remedy.
- Consider taking 400 mg of magnesium per day to relieve nervous stress and tension in your head.
- Take 5 drops of Saint-John's-wort to gain clarity and a new perspective on your health. It releases pain and tension—including migraines.
- Rub lavender oil on your temples to instantly relieve pain.

Spiritual and Energetic Solutions

- Practice spiritual vacuuming with Archangel Michael. He will take the unwanted thoughts from your mind.

- Meditate with the image of a lotus blossom. These flowers have a long history steeped in spirituality. The lotus will impart its wisdom to you by assuring you that no mistakes have ever been made. Everything has always gone the way it was Divinely meant to go.

Prayer

"Dear God and angels, please fill my head with loving thoughts and comfort. I release all tension and anxiety connected to the desire to be perfect. I know that in truth, only God is 100 percent perfect. It's okay for me to display imperfections, as my soul grows brighter with each lesson learned. Thank you."

Affirmations

- "I exchange perfection for joyful experiences."
- "I take guided action now."
- "My head is filled with loving thoughts."

Hip

Energetic Cause

You feel your foundations are unstable. You're concerned with relationships, your career, or friendships. Know that everything is going according to a higher plan, and you needn't change anything.

Natural Prescriptions

- Take 10,000 mg of good-quality flaxseed oil per day (5,000 mg twice daily). This nourishes your joints and allows freedom of movement.

- Take 2 teaspoons of corydalis for acute pain. The following day, take ½ teaspoon, in three doses throughout the day.

- Turmeric is a wonderful anti-inflammatory herb. Add it to the foods you prepare. You may also feel guided to take a turmeric supplement.

Spiritual and Energetic Solutions

- Work with Archangel Metatron's Sacred Beam of Light to clear your chakras. It may be that your root chakra is unbalanced and needs healing.

- Carry a red jasper crystal to anchor your energy and remind you that everything is stable.

- Call upon Archangel Raphael for healing intervention.

Prayer

"Dearest God, Jesus, and angels, I welcome your healing energies, and I pray for relief. Please take away all forms of pain and bless me with freedom of movement. Allow me to understand the greater plan involved. Help me to see that all is well, and everything is occurring in Divine timing. I trust you, and I surrender to this flow of energy. Thank you."

Affirmations

- "Everything is going according to a Divine plan."
- "I am safe, and all is well."
- "I trust."

Jaw

Energetic Cause

A fear of communication. You're worried that your words will cause pain to others. You're holding your tongue. Now's the time to speak the truth and share the knowledge you have.

Natural Prescriptions

- Take 7 drops of Saint-John's-wort extract to relax bodily tension and soothe your mind. It frees the muscles around your jaw and allows you to feel confident and safe.

- Take 400 mg of magnesium each day to relax tension in and around your jaw.

Spiritual and Energetic Solutions

- Sit with a bunch of daffodils, or print off a picture of them, and allow their energy to help you speak up. It's important to voice the truth; if you feel a message is important, you need to deliver it. Think of postal workers—they do not have the choice of whether or not they drop off a letter or parcel. They can't keep part and only deliver some. Everything must be given over. If you're aware of something, you need to speak up now.

- Connect with sodalite crystals; they give you confidence and also help relax the jaw.

- Release the things holding you back by performing a full-moon release ceremony.

Prayer

"Please bring healing to my jaw. I ask that this area of my body fully relax and become pain-free. Please give me the courage to speak up. Help me to choose the perfect words for every situation so that everyone benefits from what I have to say. I release fear of judgment and stand in my power to speak the truth. Thank you."

Affirmations

- "It is safe for me to speak up."
- "My words bring healing and joy."
- "Others benefit from hearing what I have to say."

Knee

Energetic Cause

You feel rushed, and you struggle to complete tasks in time. You have a sense of urgency and always feel time is running out.

Natural Prescriptions

- Start taking flaxseed oil. Begin with 3,000 mg per day, and increase to 6,000 mg if needed. Take it in divided doses, three times a day, to help the joints move freely.

- Place a cool pack on your knee in the evenings. This allows it to relax and heal.

- Consider preparing a salt pack for your knee two or three times a week. This reduces inflammation and swelling.

Spiritual and Energetic Solutions

- Meditate with a tiger's eye crystal. This heals your knee by allowing you to slow down. It is an excellent crystal for people who jump from one task to the next. Take a moment to relax and allow your body to heal.

- Place an image of baby's breath flowers underneath your pillow. This helps you better organize your time so you don't feel rushed. Baby's breath is great when you have many commitments but don't know where to start.

- Carry a fluorite crystal with you. This stone helps you relax and get some well-deserved sleep. It slows down your mind and helps you prioritize. It brings healing energy to your knee as you purposefully take the next step.

Prayer

"Dear God, Jesus, and Archangel Raphael, I call upon you now. Please send your emerald light into my knee. Please grant the healing I request as I commit to slowing down. I understand that there's no urgency; everything happens at the right time. I trust you, and I ask you to guide me on my road to recovery. Thank you."

Affirmations

- "My tasks are completed with perfect timing."
- "Today I slow down to enjoy the miracles around me."
- "I have more than enough time."

Leg

Energetic Cause

Your path is taking an unexpected change of direction. This is okay, and it's best if you go with the flow of the new path.

Natural Prescriptions

- Massage a combination of lavender and chamomile essential oils into your leg. Dilute 15 drops of each in a carrier oil—an ounce of organic olive or coconut oil. Mix well, then rub into your aching legs.

- An herb such as ginger can enhance circulation through the legs and also relieve pain. Take 20 drops three times per day in a little water.

Spiritual and Energetic Solutions

- Connect with ametrine crystals, which are excellent to carry when you are going through a phase of transition. Allow the stone to speak to you, and ask it what you can do to make this change more pleasurable.
- Let go of the past by performing a full-moon release ceremony.

Prayer

"I trust that the changes I am experiencing right now are for my highest good. I know the angels will guide me along this journey, and I confidently follow their direction. This shift is the answer to my prayers. Thank you for releasing all pain in exchange for this new experience."

Affirmations

- "I welcome positive change."
- "I allow the angels to guide me today."
- "Everything happens for a reason."

Neck

Energetic Cause

You're choosing to limit the amount you see. Do not ignore what's happening around you any longer. It's time to see things from another person's perspective.

Natural Prescriptions

- Take 12 drops of willow bark extract, four times per day, to relax the tension within your muscles.

- Take 400 mg of magnesium daily to loosen the tendons of your neck.

- Take 2 teaspoons of corydalis for acute pain. The following day, take ½ teaspoon, in three doses throughout the day.

- Take 7,000 mg of flaxseed oil in three doses each day (one dose of 3,000 mg and two doses of 2,000 mg). This will help your neck ease from side to side as you look right and left.

Spiritual and Energetic Solutions

- Work with Archangel Raphael to clear the energy of psychic attack. This negative energy often lodges itself in the delicate neck area.

- Sit in front of a tree and allow the nature angels to release your pain.

- Meditate upon the agapanthus flower. It may be a fresh blossom or a picture; both are equally effective.

This helps soften tension and uncovers more that may be going on.

- Find or purchase a small, clear quartz crystal that is double-terminated (pointed at each end). Cleanse it of old energies and program it to heal you by saying: *"Crystal, please heal my body and release all pain. I allow you to guide me in my healing as I watch for your signs. Thank you."* Using surgical tape, stick the crystal over the painful part of your neck, so one point aims at your head and the other at your feet. Leave it there for a few hours, then see if you need to repeat the process.

Prayer

"Please help me see a new perspective on my current situation. I ask that my views be flexible and relaxed as my body heals. I willingly release all pain and ask that love take its place. Angels, please bring me insights that allow me to see the bigger picture. Thank you."

Affirmations

- *"I am flexible in my views."*
- *"I am open to positive, new perspectives."*
- *"I clearly see all that goes on in my world."*

Shoulder

Energetic Cause

Carrying the weight of the world. You are burdened by the problems of others. You tend to focus on others before yourself.

Natural Prescriptions

- Take 10 drops of cramp bark three times per day to ease shoulder pain and discomfort.

- Apply a few drops of lavender or chamomile essential oil to the painful shoulder. The healing properties of the oils will reduce inflammation and take away pain.

- Consider a topical capsaicin ointment. Be cautious, as it may cause some redness. Use the smallest amount to begin with, then build up to more if needed. The capsaicin will numb the painful area, giving your shoulder relief.

Spiritual and Energetic Solutions

- Call on Archangel Michael for spiritual vacuuming. He will lift the heaviness and pain from your shoulders.

- Intuitively assess whether you need etheric cord cutting. It's likely that you help a great number of people, and every time you do so, you form an energetic cord to that individual. Ask Archangel Michael to release these unhealthy attachments so more love can flow through you.

- Clear your chakras with Archangel Metatron's Sacred Beam of Light.

- Practice regular meditation, and visualize yourself peaceful and pain-free. Take time to imagine what your life would look like if pain didn't limit you anymore.

Prayer

"Dear God and angels, please lift the weight of the world from my shoulders. I recognize that I am but one person. I am not meant to do things alone. Instead I ask you to remind me to ask for help. I welcome the healing love of my angels and the Earth Angels that surround me. Please remind me that I am not the source of people's healing. Only Heaven can create those miracles. In knowing this, I relax and enjoy the journey. Thank you."

Affirmations

- "My needs are important, and I enjoy taking care of *me.*"
- "Healing comes when the receiver is ready."
- "My shoulders move freely and comfortably."

Stomach

Energetic Cause

You bottle your emotions up. You may harbor anxiety and stress that you push down constantly.

Natural Prescriptions

- Take 10 drops of ginger tincture or liquid extract (in a little water) to relieve stomach pain and nausea.

- Try peppermint or chamomile tea to soothe your stomachache.

- Add turmeric to the foods you prepare. You may also feel guided to take a turmeric supplement.

- Rub 5 drops of chamomile essential oil onto your stomach. It will relax the area and reduce pain.

Spiritual and Energetic Solutions

- Inhale the scent of lavender essential oil to bring instant tranquillity and calm.

- Listen to the music of singing bowls, as they regulate your emotions and clear away fear.

- Use Archangel Metatron's Sacred Beam of Light to clear your chakras. He will release all anxiety and toxins that you've held on to.

Prayer

"Dear God and angels, please help me to release the pressure from within. I know it is safe for me to let go with your healing help. Please untangle the knots in my stomach so that I may find comfort once more. I ask that Archangels Michael and Raphael stand by my side and help me let go of anxiety. Thank you."

Affirmations

- "I am calm."
- "I am peaceful."
- "It is safe for me to release."

Wrist/Hand

Energetic Cause

You haven't spent enough time on the things you love. It's time to be creative and reconnect with your hobbies.

Natural Prescriptions

- Take 10 drops of ginger tincture (in a little water) to release pain and inflammation.

- Take 2.5 ml of devil's claw extract twice a day in a little water. This herb has an affinity for small joints and tendons. It will clear pain from your wrist and hands and allow you to complete the tasks ahead.

- Take 10 drops of Saint-John's-wort liquid extract for symptoms of carpal tunnel syndrome or repetitive strain injury (RSI).

- Boswellia is an excellent choice for wrist pain. Choose high-quality supplements and take the recommended dosage.

- Place a cool pack on your wrist and leave it there for 20 minutes. Let your wrist rest, then reapply the cool pack an hour later. This will reduce swelling and discomfort.

Spiritual and Energetic Solutions

- Call upon Archangel Michael and ask him to spiritually vacuum your wrist and hand. Sometimes lower energies hide in the tips of your fingers and around the tiny bones in your wrist. Archangel Michael will find them and release you from the pain.

- Hold on to a rose quartz crystal. Connect with the stone's energy and feel the vibration of love heal your wrist and hand. Initially you may sense a coolness. Then you will likely feel warmth, or tingling going through your hand and into your wrist.

- Carry a carnelian crystal with you to enhance your creative flair.

Prayer

"Dear God and angels, please give me the time, money, transportation, and anything else I may need to focus on myself. I ask you to help me rediscover my hobbies and passions. As I reacquaint myself with them, I know I will heal. Allow my joy to shine through my being and heal every muscle and joint. Thank you."

Affirmations

- "It is healing to spend time doing the things I love."
- "My creativity helps me heal."
- "I fill my time with acts of happiness."

BIBLIOGRAPHY

Abedin, L, et al. "The Effects of Dietary Alpha-linolenic Acid Compared with Docosahexaenoic Acid on Brain, Retina, Liver and Heart in the Guinea Pig," *Lipids*. 1999 May; 34(5):475–82.

Allman, MA, et al. "Supplementation with Flaxseed Oil versus Sunflower Oil in Healthy Young Men Consuming a Low Fat Diet: Effects on Platelet Composition and Function," *Eur J Clin Nutr*. 1995 Mar; 49(3):169–78.

American Academy of Pain Medicine. "AAPM Facts and Figures on Pain," accessed November 2013. www.painmed.org/patientcenter/facts_on_pain.aspx

Australian Bureau of Statistics. "Characteristics of Bodily Pain in Australia," accessed November 2013. www.abs.gov.au/ausstats/abs@.nsf/Lookup/4841.0Chapter12011

Benson, J. "Top Remedies for Treating Chronic Pain Naturally," *Natural News*, accessed November 2013. www.naturalnews.com/039092_chronic_pain_treatment _remedies.html

Bone, K. *The Ultimate Herbal Compendium*. Warwick, Queensland, Australia: Phytotherapy Press, 2007.

Buckle, J. "Use Of Aromatherapy as a Complementary Treatment for Chronic Pain," *Altern Ther Health Med*. 1999 Sep; 5(5):42–51.

Centers for Disease Control and Prevention. "About Parasites," accessed December 2013. www.cdc.gov/parasites/about.html

Centers for Disease Control and Prevention. "Policy Impact: Prescription Painkiller Overdoses," accessed November 2013. www.cdc.gov/homeandrecreationalsafety/ rxbrief

Chang HM, and PP But (eds). *Pharmacology and Applications of Chinese Materia Medica*. Singapore: World Scientific, 1987.

Davies, SJ, et al. "A Novel Treatment of Postherpetic Neuralgia Using Peppermint Oil," *Clin J Pain*. 2002 May–Jun; 18(3):200–2.

Ehrlich, S. "Devil's Claw," *University of Maryland Medical Center,* accessed November 2013. http://umm.edu/health/medical/altmed/herb/devils-claw

———. "Willow Bark," *University of Maryland Medical Center,* accessed November 2013. http://umm.edu/health/medical/altmed/herb/willow-bark

Galeotti, N, and C Ghelardini. "Saint-John's-wort Reversal of Meningeal Nociception: A Natural Therapeutic Perspective for Migraine Pain," *Phytomedicine.* 2013 Jul 15; 20(10):930–8.

Galland, L. "Intestinal Parasites May Be Causing Your Energy Slump," *The Huffington Post,* Jan 6, 2011. www.huffingtonpost.com/leo-galland-md/intestinal -parasites_b_804516.html

GNC. "MSM and the healing power of sulfur," accessed November 2013. www.gnclivewell.com.au/health-knowledge-details.asp?id=32&cid=4

Haim, J. "Treating Pain Naturally," *WellBeing,* accessed November 2013. www.wellbeing.com.au/blog/treating-pain-naturally

Henderson, JV, et al. "Prevalence, Causes, Severity, Impact, and Management of Chronic Pain in Australian General Practice Patients," *Pain Med.* 2013 Sep; 14(9):1346–61.

Institute of Medicine (IOM). *Relieving Pain in America, A Blueprint for Transforming Prevention, Care, Education, and Research.* Washington, D.C.: The National Academies Press, 2011.

Kimmatkar, N, et al. "Efficacy and Tolerability of Boswellia Serrata Extract in Treatment Of Osteoarthritis of Knee—a Randomized Double-Blind Placebo-Controlled Trial," *Phytomedicine.* 2003 Jan; 10(1):3–7.

Kizhakkedath, R. "Clinical Evaluation of a Formulation Containing Curcuma Longa and Boswellia Serrata Extracts in the Management of Knee Osteoarthritis," *Mol Med Rep.* 2013 Nov; 8(5):1542–8.

Lite, J. "Nature's New Pain Relievers," *Prevention,* November 2011. www.prevention .com/mind-body/natural-remedies/pain-remedies-11-natural-cures-pain

———. "You're in Pain. You Want Relief. Naturally," *Prevention,* September 14, 2008. www.nbcnews.com/id/26136767/ns/health-alternative_medicine/t/youre -pain-you-want-relief-naturally/#.UjkUkhY8FsM

Madhu, K, et al. "Safety and Efficacy of Curcuma Longa Extract in the Treatment of Painful Knee Osteoarthritis: A Randomized Placebo-Controlled Trial," *Inflammopharmacology.* 2013 Apr; 21(2):129–36.

Mantzioris, E, et al. "Dietary Substitution with Alpha-linolenic Acid-Rich Vegetable Oil Increases Eicosapentaenoic Acid Concentrations in Tissues," *Am J Clin Nutr.* 1994 Jun; 59(6):1304–9.

Bibliography

Mercola, J. "What you need to know about inflammation," *Mercola.com,* September 08, 2009, accessed November 2013. http://articles.mercola.com/sites/articles/archive/2009/09/08/what-you-need-to-know-about-inflammation.aspx

National Health and Medical Research Council. *Report on the Role of Polyunsaturated Fats in the Australian Diet.* Canberra: AGPS, 1991.

National Sleep Foundation. "Sleep in America Poll." 2000. www.sleepfoundation.org

Oyama, T, and G Smith (eds). *Pain and Kampo: The Use of Japanese Herbal Medicine in Management of Pain.* Tokyo: Springer-Verlag, 1994.

Paulozzi, LJ, et al. "Vital Signs: Overdoses of Prescription Opioid Pain Relievers—United States, 1999–2008," *Centers for Disease Control and Prevention.* www.cdc.gov/mmwr/preview/mmwrhtml/mm6043a4.htm

Rodriguez, T. "Common Parasite Linked to Personality Changes," *Scientific American,* Aug 2, 2012, accessed December 2013, www.scientificamerican.com/article.cfm?id=common-parasite-linked-to-personality-changes

Schmid, B, et al. "Efficacy and Tolerability of a Standardized Willow Bark Extract in Patients with Osteoarthritis: Results of Two Randomized Double-Blind Controlled Studies," *Phytother Res.* 2001; 15: 344–350.

Substance Abuse and Mental Health Services Administration. *Drug Abuse Warning Network: Selected Tables of National Estimates of Drug-Related Emergency Department Visits.* Rockville, MD: Substance Abuse and Mental Health Services Administration, 2010.

———. *Results from the 2010 National Survey on Drug Use and Health: Summary of National Findings.* NSDUH Series H-41, HHS Publication No. (SMA) 11-4658. Rockville, MD: Substance Abuse and Mental Health Services Administration, 2011. http://oas.samhsa.gov/NSDUH/2k10NSDUH/2k10Results.htm

Thomsen, M. *Phytotherapy Desk Reference.* Tasmania: Global Natural Medicine, 2005.

Virtue, D. *The Healing Miracles of Archangel Raphael.* Carlsbad, CA: Hay House, 2011.

☙ ❧

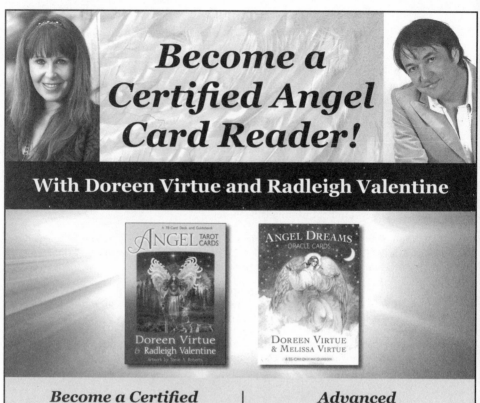

ABOUT THE AUTHORS

Doreen Virtue holds Ph.D., M.A., and B.A. degrees in counseling psychology, and she is the daughter of a professional spiritual healer. Doreen grew up with prayer healing every ache and pain in her family. She wrote about healing pain in her book *The Healing Miracles of Archangel Raphael*. She has appeared on *Oprah,* CNN, *The View, Coast to Coast AM,* and many other TV and radio programs. Doreen gives workshops worldwide and online on HayHouseRadio.com.

To learn more about Doreen's work and products, please visit: AngelTherapy.com or facebook.com/DoreenVirtue444.

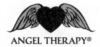

ANGEL THERAPY®

Robert Reeves, N.D., is an accredited naturopath who blends his herbal medicine and nutrition training with his psychic and mediumship abilities. He has a strong connection to the angels and to the natural world, believing that nature holds Divine healing properties.

Robert teaches spiritual workshops, writes magazine articles, and has been featured on international radio programs. He owns and runs a successful natural-therapies clinic in Australia, where he has assisted numerous clients in healing from pain. He has developed a range of vibrational essences focusing on crystal and angel energy, which are currently available as aura sprays. Robert is co-author, with Doreen, of *Flower Therapy, Flower Therapy Oracle Cards,* and *Angel Detox.*

For more information about Robert, please visit: www.Robert Reeves.com.au or facebook.com/RobertReevesNaturopath.

Hay House Titles of Related Interest

YOU CAN HEAL YOUR LIFE, the movie, starring Louise Hay & Friends
(available as a 1-DVD program and an expanded 2-DVD set)
Watch the trailer at: www.LouiseHayMovie.com

THE SHIFT, the movie,
starring Dr. Wayne W. Dyer
(available as a 1-DVD program and an expanded 2-DVD set)
Watch the trailer at: www.DyerMovie.com

☙

LOVING YOURSELF TO GREAT HEALTH: Thoughts & Food—the Ultimate Diet, by Louise Hay, Ahlea Khadro, and Heather Dane

MEALS THAT HEAL INFLAMMATION: Embrace Healthy Living and Eliminate Pain, One Meal at a Time, by Julie Daniluk, R.H.N.

ONE MIND: How Our Individual Mind Is Part of a Greater Consciousness and Why It Matters, by Larry Dossey, M.D.

STOP PAIN: Inflammation Relief for an Active Life, by Vijay Vad, M.D.

All of the above are available at your local bookstore,
or may be ordered by contacting Hay House (see next page).

☙

We hope you enjoyed this Hay House book. If you'd like to receive our online catalog featuring additional information on Hay House books and products, or if you'd like to find out more about the Hay Foundation, please contact:

Hay House, Inc., P.O. Box 5100, Carlsbad, CA 92018-5100
(760) 431-7695 or (800) 654-5126
(760) 431-6948 (fax) or (800) 650-5115 (fax)
www.hayhouse.com® • www.hayfoundation.org

🙢

Published and distributed in Australia by: Hay House Australia Pty. Ltd., 18/36 Ralph St., Alexandria NSW 2015 • *Phone:* 612-9669-4299 • *Fax:* 612-9669-4144 www.hayhouse.com.au

Published and distributed in the United Kingdom by: Hay House UK, Ltd., Astley House, 33 Notting Hill Gate, London W11 3JQ • *Phone:* 44-20-3675-2450 *Fax:* 44-20-3675-2451 • www.hayhouse.co.uk

Published and distributed in the Republic of South Africa by: Hay House SA (Pty), Ltd., P.O. Box 990, Witkoppen 2068 • *Phone/Fax:* 27-11-467-8904 www.hayhouse.co.za

Published in India by: Hay House Publishers India, Muskaan Complex, Plot No. 3, B-2, Vasant Kunj, New Delhi 110 070 • *Phone:* 91-11-4176-1620 *Fax:* 91-11-4176-1630 • www.hayhouse.co.in

Distributed in Canada by: Raincoast Books, 2440 Viking Way, Richmond, B.C. V6V 1N2 • *Phone:* 1-800-663-5714 • *Fax:* 1-800-565-3770 • www.raincoast.com

🙢

Take Your Soul on a Vacation

Visit www.HealYourLife.com® to regroup, recharge, and reconnect with your own magnificence. Featuring blogs, mind-body-spirit news, and life-changing wisdom from Louise Hay and friends.

Visit www.HealYourLife.com today!

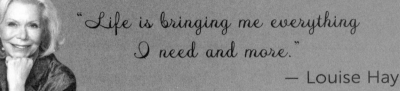